Trocar Surgery for Cataract Surgeons

Ulrich Spandau

Trocar Surgery for Cataract Surgeons

From Dislocated IOL to Dropped Nucleus

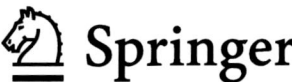 Springer

Ulrich Spandau
Department of Ophthalmology
Uppsala University Hospital
Uppsala
Uppsala Län
Sweden

ISBN 978-3-030-36092-4   ISBN 978-3-030-36093-1   (eBook)
https://doi.org/10.1007/978-3-030-36093-1

This Springer imprint is published by the registered company Springer Nature Switzerland AG
The registered company address is: Gewerbestrasse 11, 6330 Cham, Switzerland

This book is dedicated to my wife Katrin

Preface

Trocar surgery has revolutionized vitrectomy in the last 10 years. I am convinced that trocars will also revolutionize anterior segment surgery because trocars conquer the pars plana region for cataract surgeons. Trocars are easy to use, they are easy to insert, and the usage of instruments through trocar cannulas is simple.

The conquest of the pars plana opens a completely new field of possible anterior segment surgeries which were prior reserved for vitreoretinal surgeons. For example, a dislocated IOL can be retrieved easily from pars plana and elevated into the anterior chamber; this maneuver, however, is difficult from the limbus Or in case of positive vitreous pressure during cataract surgery an anterior vitrectomy from pars plana can relieve the pressure. Furthermore, anterior vitrectomy from pars plana secondary to posterior capsular rupture or an anterior vitrectomy from pars plana for vitreous prolapse secondary to zonular lysis is also possible.

An anterior vitrectomy from pars plana is easier from pars plana than from the limbus because the lens capsule is not in the way. The anterior vitreous can be removed completely reducing the risk of postoperative vitreous prolapse and reducing the risk of injuring the lens capsule.

Last but not least this book will show the surgery of a dropped nucleus with a cataract machine. This technique was pioneered in Uppsala, Sweden, and is very easy to reproduce. With a phacoemulsification machine and a regular phacoemulsification handpiece, a removal of a dropped nucleus is possible.

I am convinced that anterior and posterior segment surgery will fuse in the future. The modern cataract machines have a powerful vitrectomy function and in case of a dropped nucleus a cataract surgeon can convert with the same machine to a vitrectomy and remove the nucleus.

The book includes many videos, which demonstrate the surgeries step by step. If you have the hardcover version of the book, you can view the videos on my youtube channel. If you have the online version of the book or e-book, you can view the video by clicking on the doi link. The doi link can be found on the first page of each chapter.

Uppsala, Sweden   Ulrich Spandau

Acknowledgements

I want to thank my colleagues, Dr Samanta and Dr Majumdar and especially Dr Sanyal, for proofreading my manuscript and giving valuable suggestions for improvement.

Contents

Abbreviations

CPM	Cuts per minute
I / A	Irrigation and aspiration
ECCE	Extracapsular cataract extraction
G	Gauge
ICCE	Intracapsular cataract extraction
IOL	Intraocular lens
in-the-bag IOL	Intraocular lens is located inside the lens capsule
PCO	Posterior capsular opacification
PMMA	Polymethylmethacrylate (=plexiglas)
PPV	Pars plana vitrectomy
PCR	Posterior capsular rent (rupture)
PVD	Posterior vitreous detachment
SICS	Manual Small incision cataract surgery (=modified ECCE)
Viscoelastics	Provisc®, Duovisc®, Viscoat® (not HPMC)

List of Videos

The following videos can be accessed under my youtube channel. If you have the online version of the book or e-book, you can also view the video by clicking on the doi link.

The doi link can be found on the first page of each chapter.

Part I
Introduction to Trocar Surgery

Chapter 1
What Is Trocar Surgery?

Trocars have been introduced in 2003 and have revolutionized vitrectomy. Trocar cannulas consist of a metal cannula and a plug (valve) (Fig. 1.1). The trocar cannulas are inserted in the sclera and protect the surrounding tissue from the repeated insertion of instruments. The valves prevent fluid loss through the trocar cannulas and maintain a water tight globe.

The trocars allow the anterior segment surgeon to access the pars plana which was prior reserved to posterior segment surgeons. The borders of the cataract surgeon are expanded from the posterior lens capsule to pars plana; and the conquest of the pars plana extends the surgical spectrum of an anterior segment surgeon immensely.

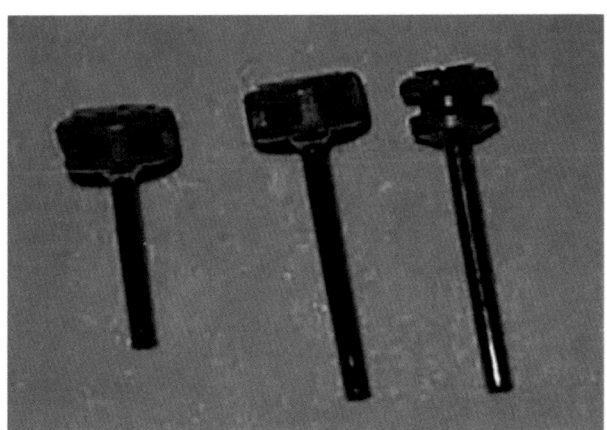

Fig. 1.1 23 Gauge trocar cannula. A trocar cannula consists of a metal cannula and a (orange) plug (valve). The latter prevents outflow of intraocular fluid

© Springer Nature Switzerland AG 2020
U. Spandau, *Trocar Surgery for Cataract Surgeons*,
https://doi.org/10.1007/978-3-030-36093-1_1

1.1   Possible Indications for Trocar Surgery of Anterior Segment

Possible indications for trocar surgery of anterior segment are:

1. Anterior vitrectomy secondary to posterior capsular rent (Figs. 1.2 and 1.3).
2. Vitreous prolapse secondary to zonular lysis (Fig. 1.4).
3. Cortical material behind the lens capsule (Fig. 1.5).

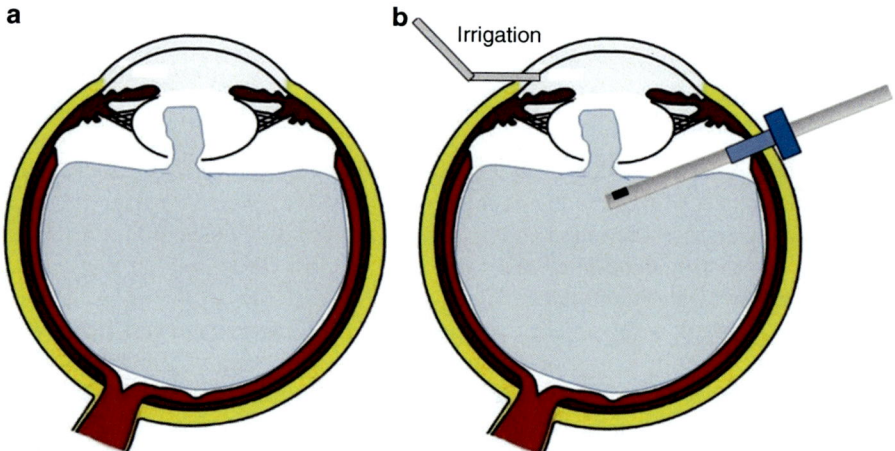

Fig. 1.2 Anterior vitrectomy secondary to posterior capsular rent: (**a**) A posterior capsular rent with vitreous prolapse. (**b**) An anterior vitrectomy from pars plana allows a safe removal of anterior vitreous because the risk to injure the lens capsule is reduced

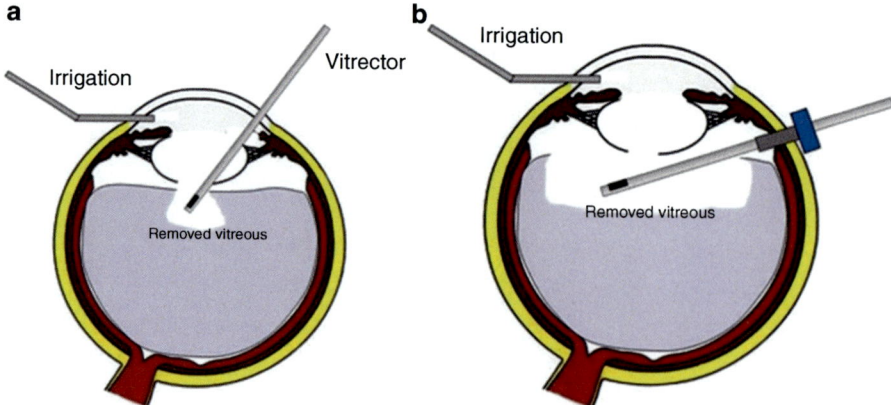

Fig. 1.3 Conventional anterior vitrectomy versus anterior vitrectomy from pars plana: (**a**) The conventional anterior vitrectomy allows only a partial removal of anterior vitreous because the lens capsule and the iris are in the way. (**b**) In contrast, the anterior vitrectomy from pars plana allows a complete removal of the anterior vitreous because of better accessibility

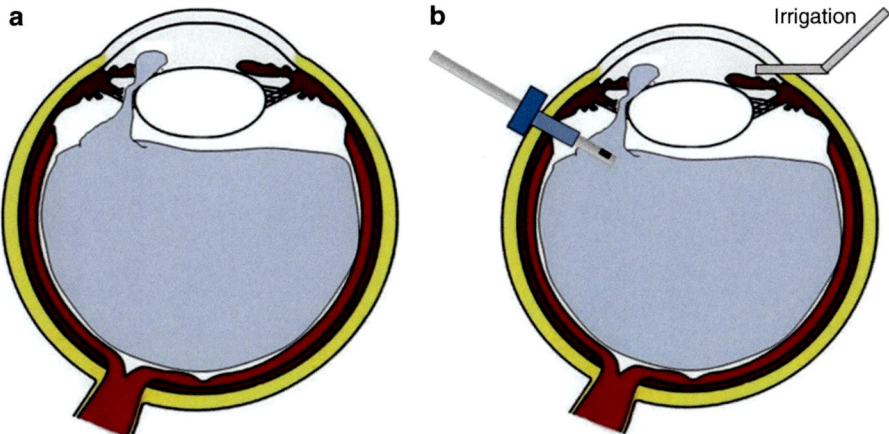

Fig. 1.4 Vitreous prolapse secondary to zonular lysis: (**a**) This pathology cannot be solved in a conventional way with anterior vitrectomy from the limbus because the iris comes in the way. (**b**) Only from pars plana you can access the anterior vitreous and remove the prolapse

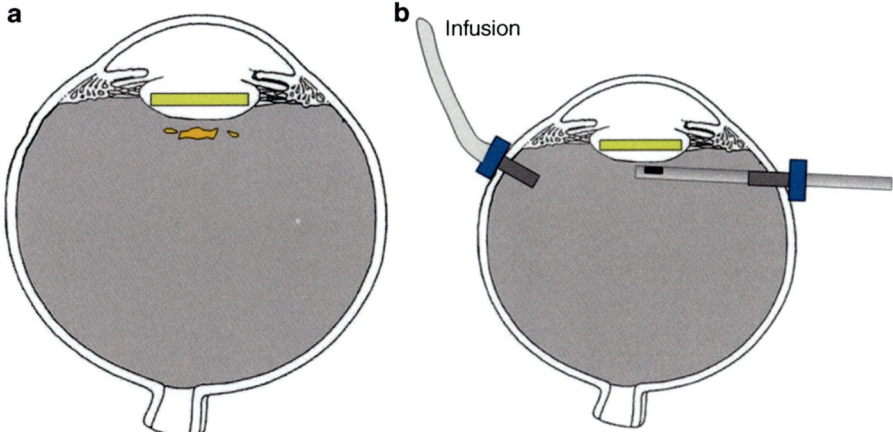

Fig. 1.5 Dropped cortical material secondary to zonular lysis or posterior capsular rent: (**a**) The IOL is located in the bag and the cortical material is located directly behind the lens capsule. This pathology cannot be solved in a conventional way with anterior vitrectomy from the limbus. (**b**) Only from pars plana you can remove completely the cortical fragments

4. Positive vitreous pressure during cataract surgery (Fig. 1.6).
5. Removal of posterior capsular opacification from pars plana (Fig. 1.7).
6. Subluxated IOL (Fig. 1.8).
7. Dropping nucleus (Fig. 1.9).

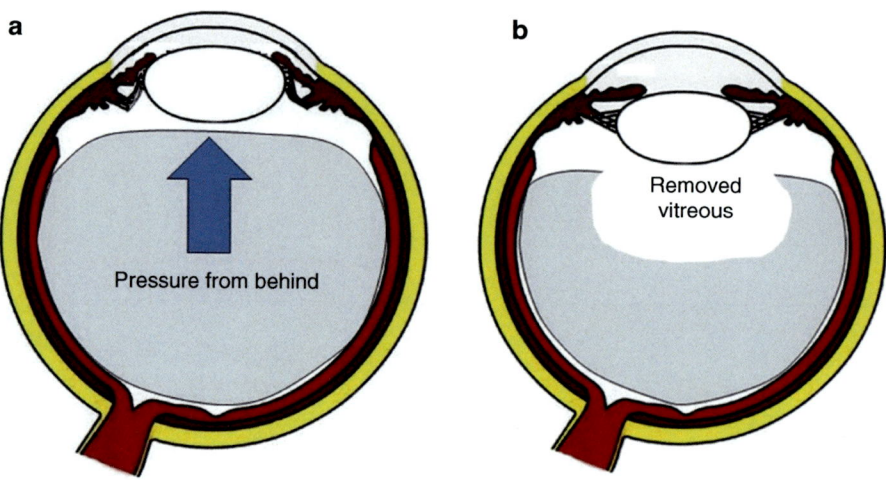

Fig. 1.6 Positive vitreous pressure during cataract surgery: (**a**) The lens-iris diaphragm is pressed towards the cornea making further surgery impossible. (**b**) Remove the anterior vitreous from pars plana and the iris-lens diaphragm regain its normal position

Fig. 1.7 Removal of posterior capsular opacification from pars plana: A PCO can be easily removed from pars plana. Possible candidates are patients who are unable to position behind the slit lamp for YAG laser, thick PCO's or children

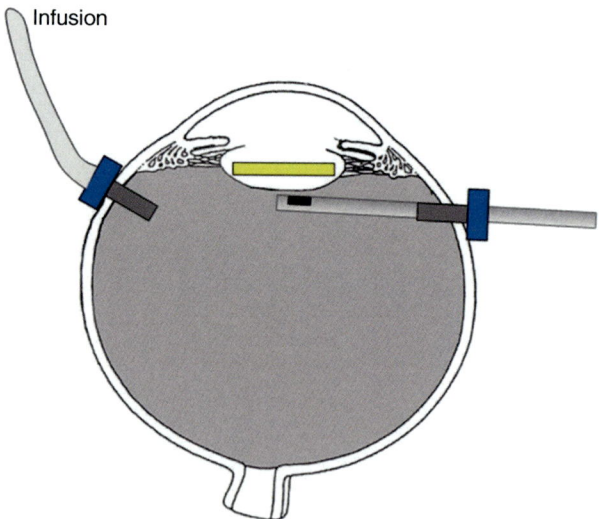

1.2   Possible Indications for Trocar Surgery of Posterior Segment

Trocar surgery must not be limited to the pars plana and anterior vitreous. If you purchase a viewing system and a light source, you can operate all through out in the posterior segment. Posterior segment consists of anterior and posterior vitreous.

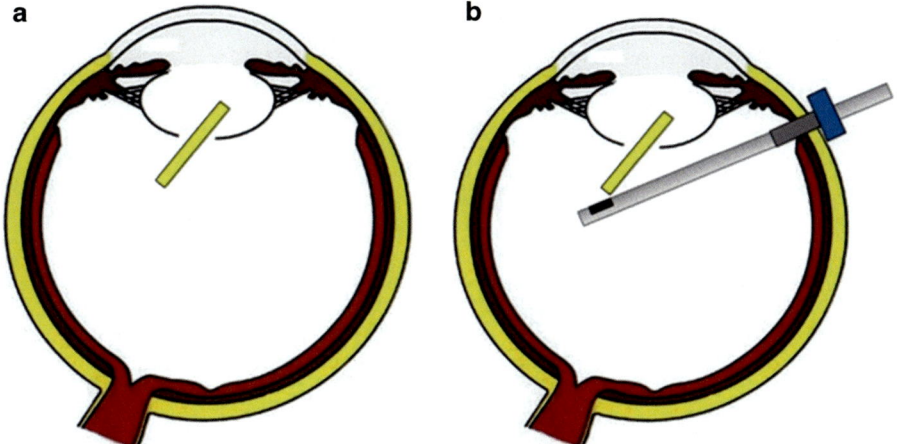

Fig. 1.8 Subluxated IOL: (**a**) The recovery of a subluxated IOL is difficult and in the most cases impossible from the limbus. (**b**) From pars plana the recovery is easy. Insert an instrument at pars plana and lift the IOL into the anterior chamber

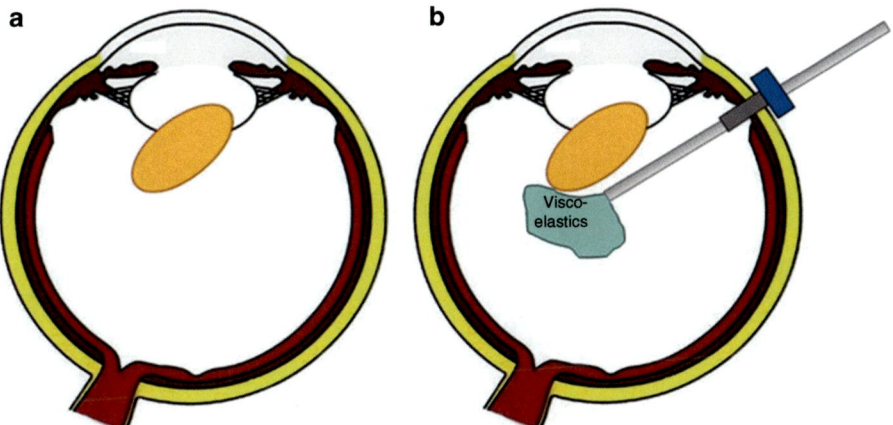

Fig. 1.9 (**a**) The nucleus is dropping due to PCR: (**b**) Introduce a viscoelastics cannula at pars plana, inject viscoelastics (Viscoat®) behind the nucleus and then elevate it into the anterior chamber

When you mean to operate in the posterior vitreous, it is better to say all through out in posterior segment or in posterior vitreous. A vitrectomy machine is not required, a phacoemulsification machine is sufficient. The possible indications for trocar surgery of posterior segment are:

1. Dropped nucleus (Fig. 1.10).
2. Posterior dislocated IOL (Fig. 1.11).

Fig. 1.10 Dropped
nucleus: The nucleus has
dropped onto the retina. A
vitrectomy is required.
This is possible with a
phacoemulsification
machine

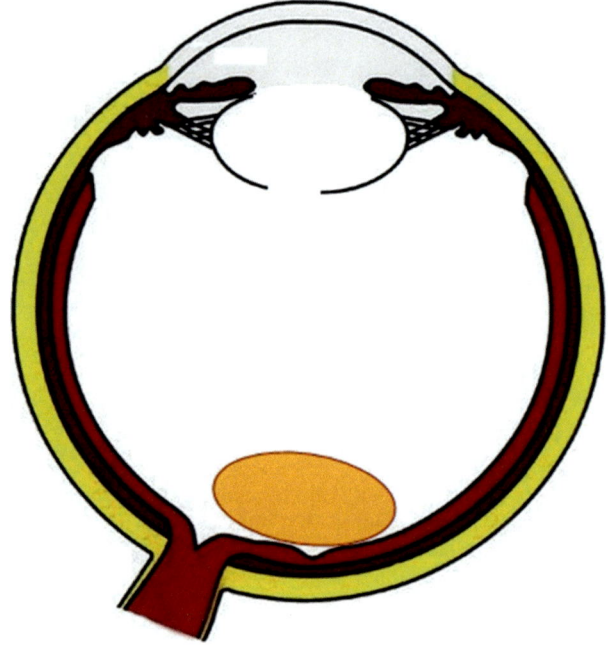

Fig. 1.11 Posterior
dislocated IOL: The IOL
has luxated onto the
posterior pole. A
vitrectomy is required.
Even this surgery is
possible with a
phacoemulsification
machine

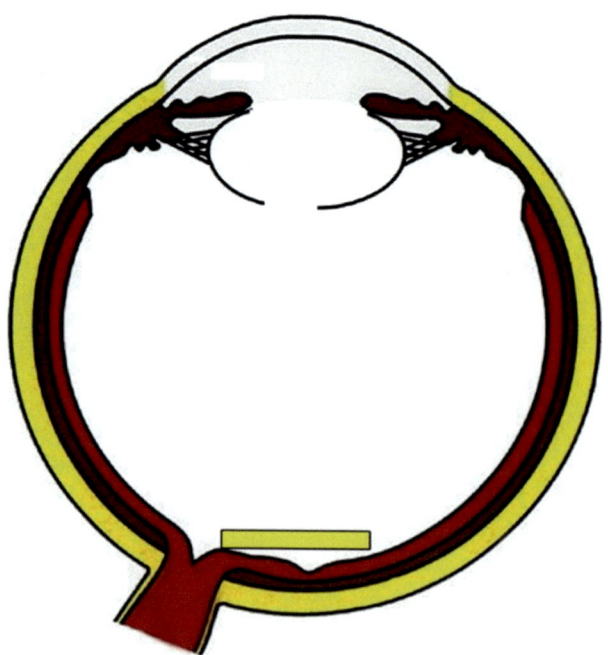

1.3   Advantages of Anterior Vitrectomy with Trocar Cannulas from Pars Plana

For the conventional anterior vitrectomy, a vitreous cutter is inserted through a corneal incision and the vitreous behind the lens capsule is removed. The removal of the anterior vitreous is, however, limited to the size of the posterior capsular rent. In the most cases the PCR allows only a partial removal of the anterior vitreous (Fig. 1.12). This results often in a postoperative vitreous prolapse.

An *incomplete* removal of the anterior vitreous occurs often after an anterior vitrectomy from the limbus. Postoperatively, it often results in a vitreous prolapse in the anterior chamber or a vitreous strand towards a corneal incision causing a traction on the retina (Fig. 1.13). After several months this traction may result in a retinal detachment.

In contrast, an anterior vitrectomy from pars plana takes place behind the lens capsule. A complete removal of the anterior vitreous is possible because the lens capsule and the iris are no longer in way (Fig. 1.14). A postoperative vitreous prolapse is unlikely. In addition, the risk to damage the lens capsule during vitrectomy is low.

Fig. 1.12 Anterior vitrectomy from the anterior chamber. Only a small part of the anterior vitreous can be removed. In addition, the risk to damage the remaining lens capsule is high. This insufficient removal results often in a postoperative vitreous prolapse

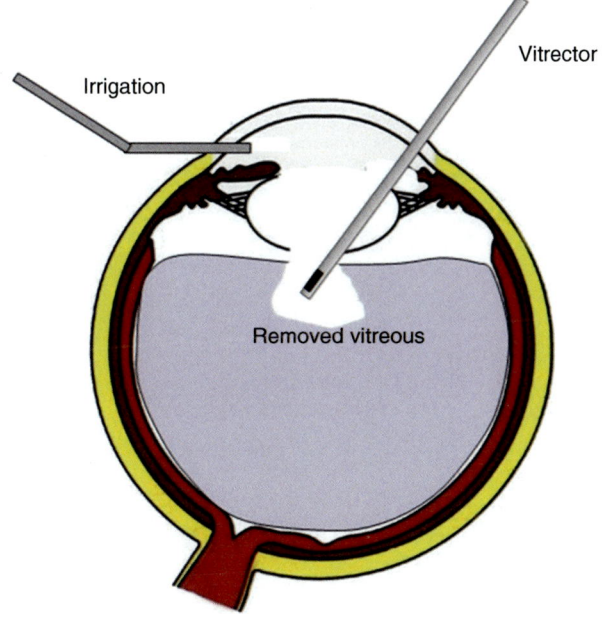

Irrigation

Vitrector

Removed vitreous

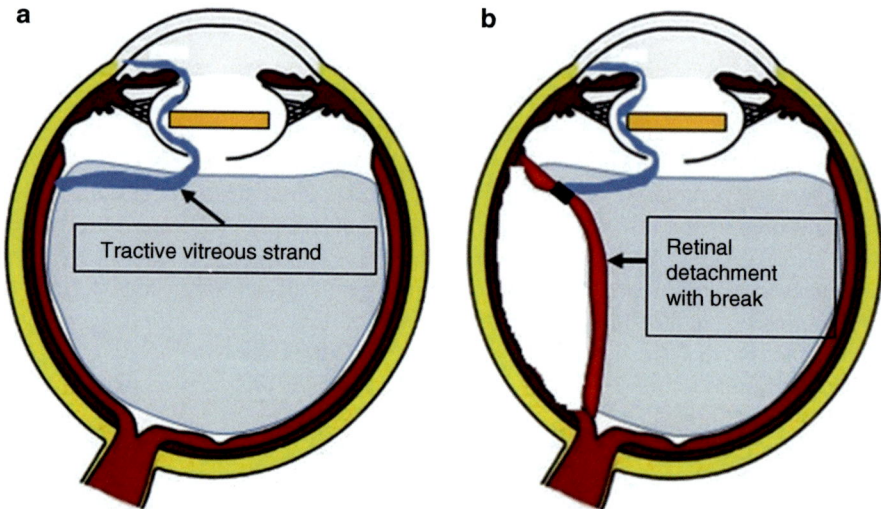

Fig. 1.13 (**a**) A vitreous strand causes traction on the retina. (**b**) After several months the traction may cause a retinal detachment

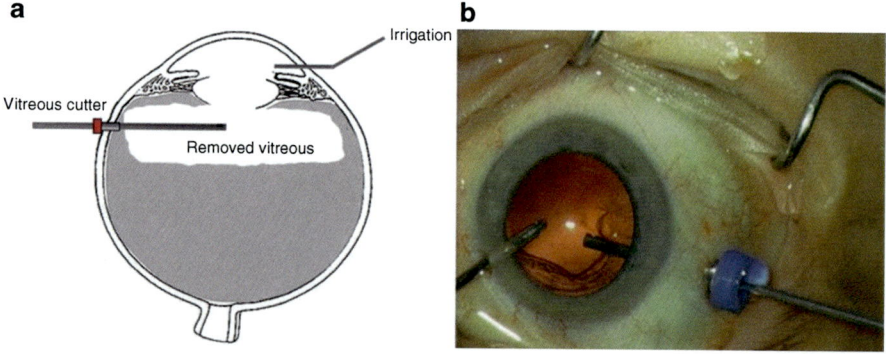

Fig. 1.14 Anterior vitrectomy from pars plana. The anterior vitreous can be removed to 100% (**a**) and there is no risk to damage the lens capsule (**b**)

Part II
Equipment and Fundamentals
About Trocar Surgery

Chapter 2
Equipment for Surgery of Anterior Segment

The Video 2.1 demonstrates the basics and the setup of a vitreous cutter.

The required equipment for trocar surgery of anterior segment is as follows:

1. Phacoemulsification machine, Fig. 2.1
2. Anterior vitreous cutter (23G), Figs. 2.2 and 2.3
3. Trocars (23G), Figs. 2.4 and 2.5
4. Infusion line (23G), Fig. 2.6

Phacoemulsification Machines

You can use any modern phacoemulsification machine, Infinity (Alcon), Centurion (Alcon), Stellaris (B&L), all of them have powerful anterior vitreous cutters (Fig. 2.1). The cutting frequency of an anterior vitreous cutter for *Alcon Infinity* is 2500 cpm (cuts per minute), for *Alcon Centurion* 4000 cpm and for *Bausch & Lomb Stellaris* 5000 cpm. For the *Oertli Catarex 3* the cutting rate is 1200 cuts/min but the cutter cuts both ways, while going forward and backward, resulting in 2400 cpm. The Gauge of the anterior vitreous cutter is 23G (Fig. 2.2). There is no anterior vitreous cutter for 25G or 27G available. You can also use other phacoemulsification machines. The essential point is that the anterior vitreous cutter should be 23 Gauge and not 20 Gauge because there are no trocars available for 20 Gauge. There are only trocars available for 23 Gauge. In short, if your phacoemulsification machine has a 23 Gauge anterior vitreous cutter then you can perform all surgeries mentioned in this book.

Anterior Vitreous Cutter (Video 2.1)

The *old* vitreous cutters were coaxial; i.e. the cutter was combined with irrigation. The *modern* cutters are not coaxial and have, therefore, *no* irrigation. Anterior vitreous cutter are pneumatic vitreous cutters meaning that the port opening and closing

Electronic Supplementary Material The online version of this chapter (https://doi.org/10.1007/978-3-030-36093-1_2) contains supplementary material, which is available to authorized users.

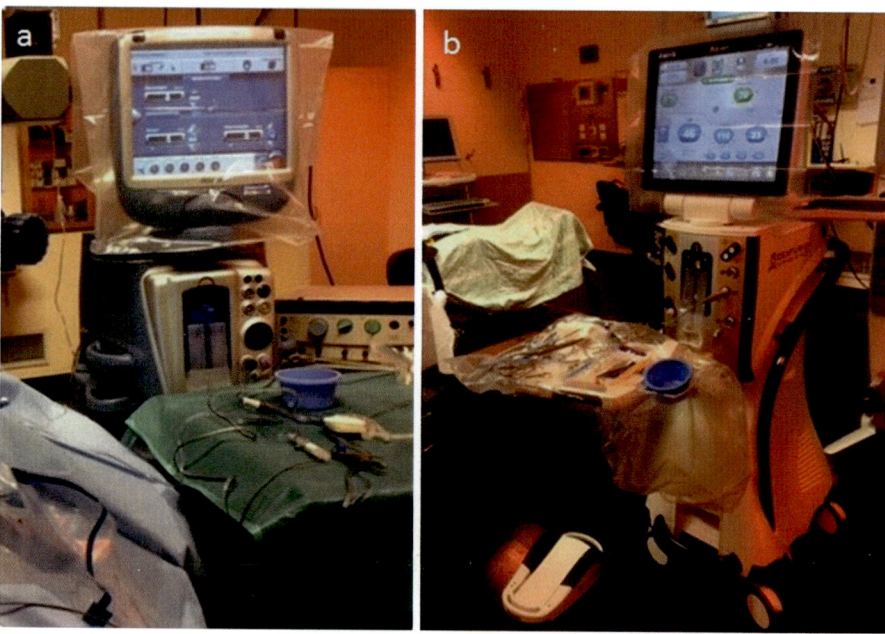

Fig. 2.1 Infinity machine (**a**) and Centurion machine (**b**). All modern phacoemulsification machines have a 23G anterior vitreous cutter

Fig. 2.2 Anterior vitreous cutter (23G) from Alcon. Anterior vitreous cutters come in two sizes, 20 Gauge and 23 Gauge. All modern anterior vitreous cutters are 23G

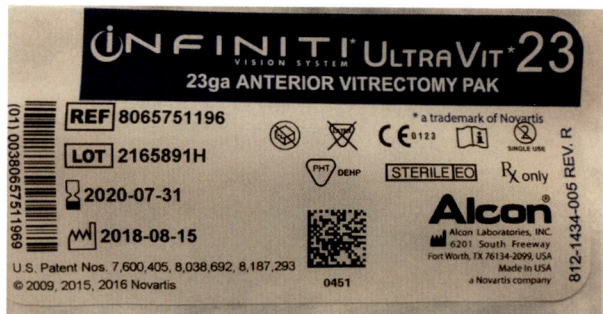

is controlled by air. Pneumatic spring cutters have two tubings, one tubing steers the cutting and the second is for aspiration. The dual pneumatic vitreous cutters from Alcon has three tubings, one for the aspiration and two for the dual-pneumatic drive (Figs. 2.2 and 2.3). The two tubings for the pneumatic drive are connected to the phacoemulsification machine. These tubes steer the opening and closing of the port of the vitreous cutter. The third tubing is connected to the aspiration port of the phacoemulsification machine and aspirates the fluid from the eye. There is *no* irrigation inside the cutter. The vitreous cutter aspirates fluid from the eye but does *not* irrigate the eye. Therefore, a separate irrigation handpiece is required to replace the aspirated fluid and maintain the IOP in the eye.

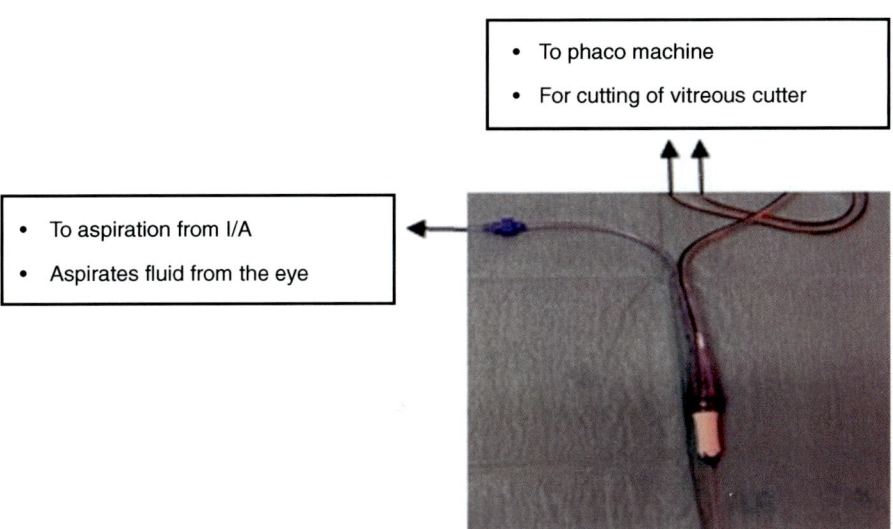

• To phaco machine

• For cutting of vitreous cutter

• To aspiration from I/A

• Aspirates fluid from the eye

Fig. 2.3 Three tubings are connected to the vitreous cutter. Two tubings are connected to the phacoemulsification machine. They steer the cutting function of the vitreous cutter. The third (blue) tubing is attached to the aspiration tube of I/A. This tubing aspirates the fluid from the vitreous cutter and transports it to the cassette. Remark: There is no irrigation inside the vitreous cutter. Irrigation is maintained by an irrigation handpiece or an infusion line

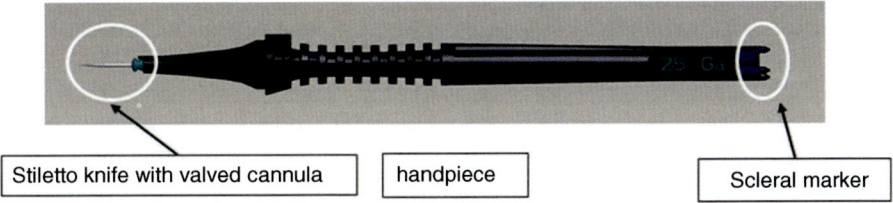

Stiletto knife with valved cannula   handpiece   Scleral marker

Fig. 2.4 A trocar. On the left side is the stiletto knife with valve. In the middle is the handpiece. On the right side is the scleral marker which marks the distance from the limbus

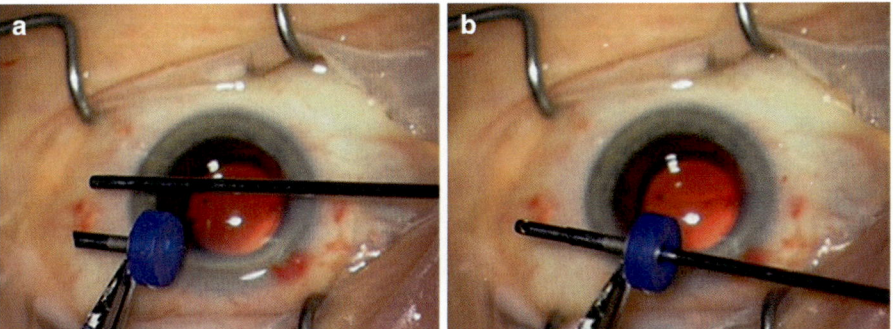

Fig. 2.5 (**a**) A trocar with blue valve (DORC) and a vitreous cutter. (**b**) The blue valve prevents outflow of intraocular fluid

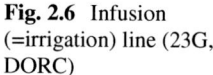

Fig. 2.6 Infusion
(=irrigation) line (23G,
DORC)

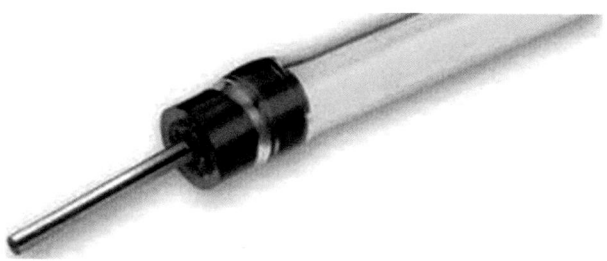

Caution A vitrectomy without irrigation results in an under pressure of the globe. The choroidal vessels are injured and a dangerous subchoroidal hemorrhage with malignant glaucoma develops.

Trocars

Trocars are simple to use. A trocar has a trocar handpiece which consists of a stiletto knife and a valved cannula. Behind the handpiece is a scleral marker All modern 23G trocars include a handpiece, a knife with trocar and a marker (Fig. 2.4). Trocars are available from many companies. Trocar cannulas facilitate the insertion of instruments and protect the surrounding tissue. The valves prevent the outflow from intraocular fluid keeping the globe normotone (Fig. 2.5).

Anterior vitreous cutters of 23 G need to be used as it is compatible with 23 G trocars. You can purchase 23G trocars of any company, they can all be used with a 23G vitreous cutter (Fig. 2.5).

For trocar surgery you need at least one 23G trocar. This trocar is used for the vitreous cutter. It is, however, better and easier to work with two trocars. The second trocar can be used for the infusion line (Fig. 2.6). The infusion line replaces the irrigation handpiece. For the most surgeries 1–2 trocars are sufficient.

The trocars and infusion line are available as a kit from the following companies (Figs. 2.7, 2.8, 2.9, 2.10).

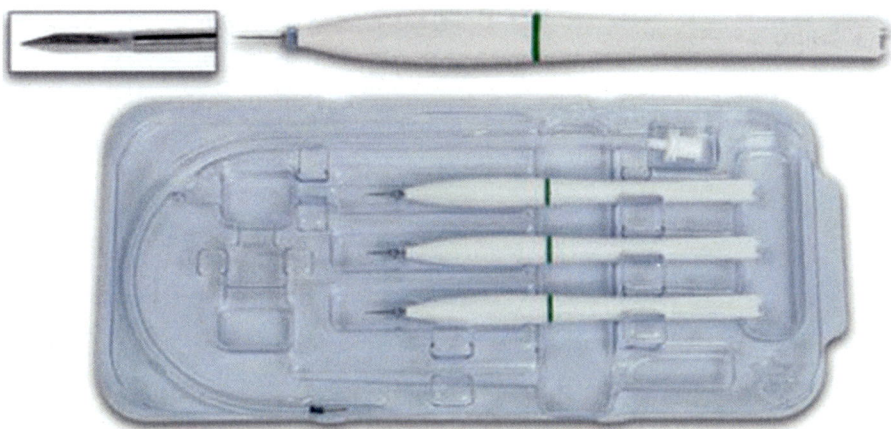

Fig. 2.7 23G trocar from DORC No: 1272.ED206. This package includes three trocars and one infusion line (DORC, NL). Remark: DORC manufactures one step disposable valved 23 G trocars

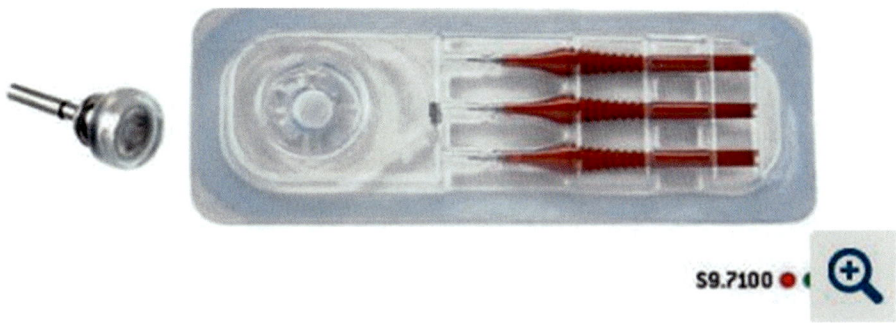

S9.7100

Fig. 2.8 This package includes three 23G trocars and one infusion (irrigation) line. (FCI, France No. S9.7100.23)

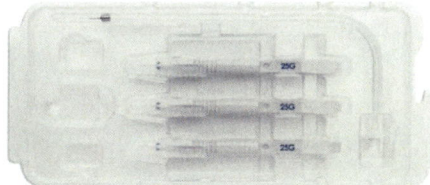

Product Name	Packaging	Order #
Trocar Kit 25G S	3 Kits / Box	MTK25S
Trocar Kit 23G S	3 Kits / Box	MTK23S

• Sterile 1 Kit consists of 3 pcs. trocar with the valved cannula and 1 pc. infusion cannula.

Fig. 2.9 This package includes three 23G trocars and one infusion (irrigation) line. (Mani, Japan MTK23S)

Fig. 2.10 This package includes three 23G trocars and one infusion (irrigation) line. (Aurolab, India)

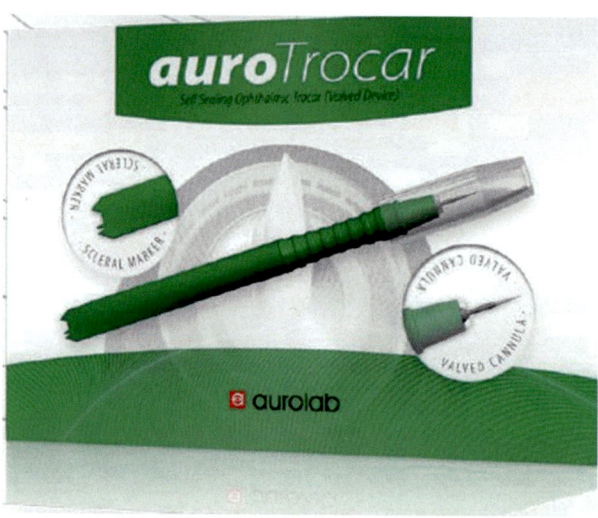

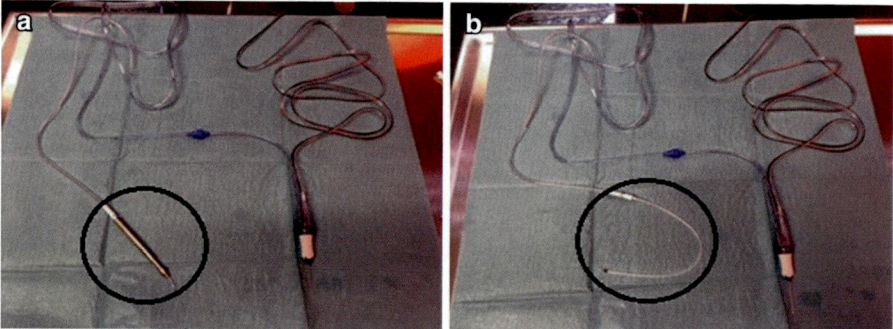

Fig. 2.11 (**a**) Conventional setup of anterior vitreous cutter with irrigation handpiece (circle). (**b**) Novel setup of vitreous cutter with infusion line for trocar surgery (circle)

2.1   Setup of Anterior Vitreous Cutter

In the conventional setup, the anterior vitreous cutter is used with an irrigation handpiece (Fig. 2.11a). Remember that the new vitreous cutters are non-coaxial. In trocar surgery, the irrigation handpiece is replaced by an infusion line (Fig. 2.11b). This infusion is included in the aforementioned packages (Figs. 2.7, 2.8, 2.9, 2.10)

Chapter 3
Setup and Basics About Trocar Surgery

The setup of the anterior vitreous cutter is very simple. Attach the two main tubings in the phaco machine and the short tubing to the aspiration tube from I/A (Fig. 3.1). If you want to perform an anterior vitrectomy with one trocar then attach an irrigation cannula or irrigation handpiece (Fig. 3.1). If you want to perform an anterior vitrectomy with two trocars, then attach an infusion line to the irrigation tube (Fig. 3.1).

Remark: Avoid the old coaxial vitreous cutters. Coaxial means irrigation and vitrectomy in one handpiece. A coaxial vitreous cutter hydrates the vitreous and causes further prolapse.

There are three possible setups for the irrigation:

1. Irrigation handpiece in anterior chamber (Fig. 3.2a).

The *advantage* is that it is easy to use, and the *disadvantage* is that you have no free hand.

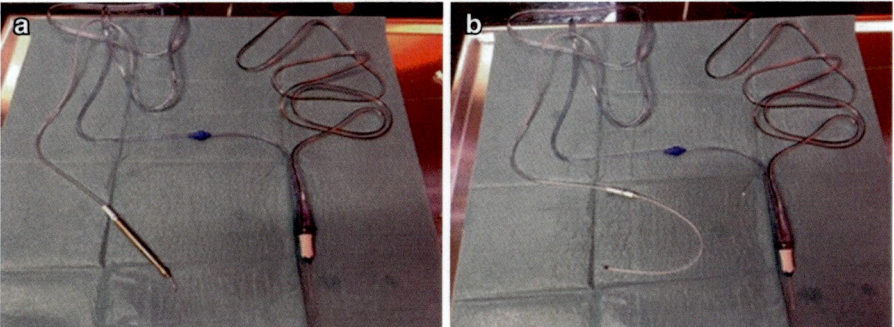

Fig. 3.1 (**a**) Conventional setup of anterior vitreous cutter. This is also the setup for trocar surgery with one trocar. (**b**) Novel setup of vitreous cutter with infusion (irrigation) line for trocar surgery with two trocars

Electronic supplementary material The online version of this chapter (https://doi.org/10.1007/978-3-030-36093-1_3) contains supplementary material, which is available to authorized users.

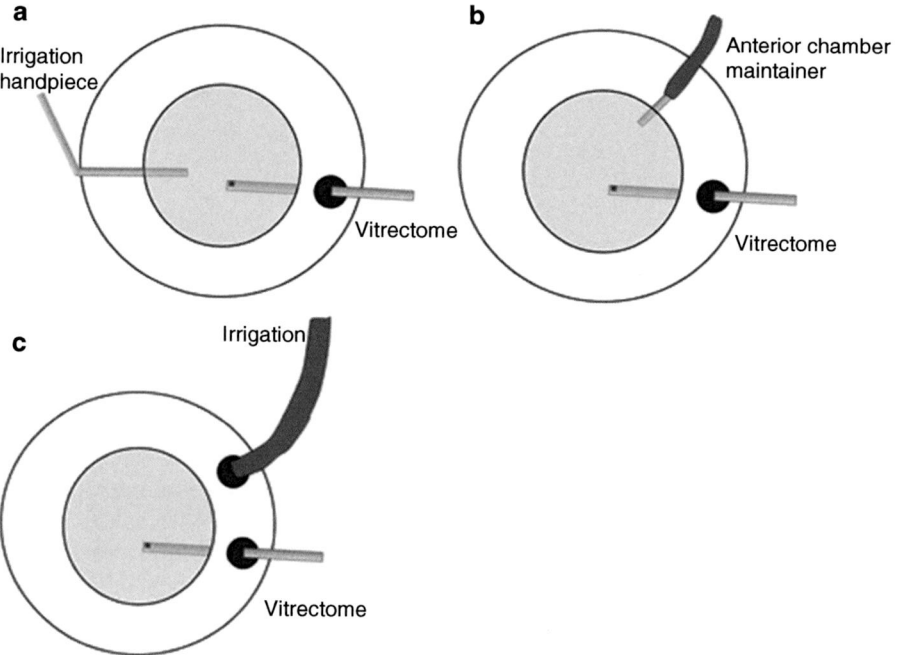

Fig. 3.2 (**a**) Conventional technique for anterior vitreous cutter with an irrigation handpiece in anterior chamber. (**b**) An alternative is the insertion of an anterior chamber maintainer. (**c**) The best technique is an infusion from pars plana. A second trocar cannula is inserted in the pars plana. The infusion line is inserted into the trocar cannula providing a stable infusion

2. Anterior chamber maintainer in anterior chamber (Fig. 3.2b).

The *advantage* is that you have a free hand, and the *disadvantage* is that the infusion is unstable and dislocates easily.

3. Trocar cannula in pars plana (Fig. 3.2c).

The *advantage* is that you have a free hand and the infusion is stable and does not dislocate. Also you are exposing the cornea endothelium less to direct irrigation from fluids as your infusion is away from the cornea. There is no *disadvantage*.

3.1   Trocar Surgery with One Trocar

Trocar surgery with one trocar is very simple (see Video 3.1). The setup of the vitreous cutter is identical as if you work without trocar; the infusion line is attached to the irrigation handpiece (Fig. 3.3). One trocar is inserted into the sclera on the temporal side (Fig. 3.4a). The vitreous cutter is inserted through this trocar and the

Fig. 3.3 The conventional
setup for anterior
vitrectomy with an Alcon
machine. On the right side
you see the anterior
vitreous cutter and on the
left side the irrigation
handpiece

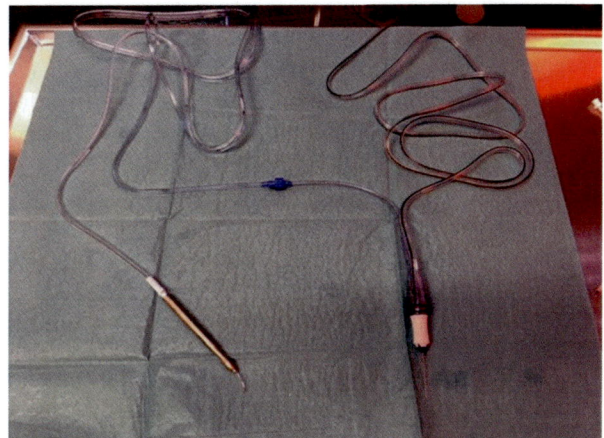

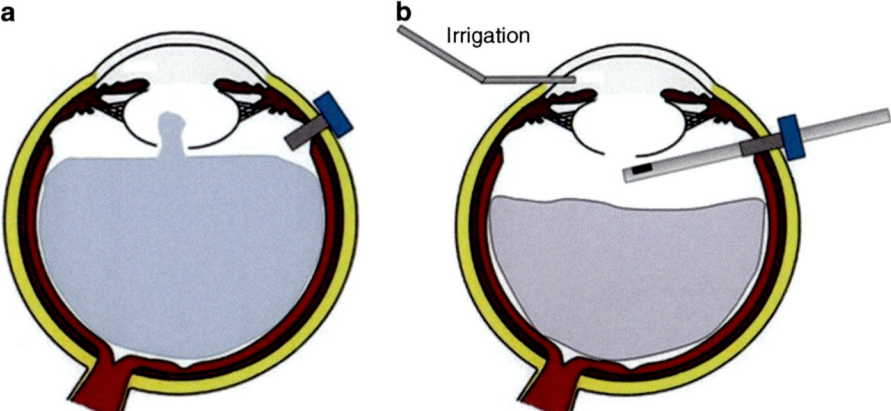

Fig. 3.4 (**a**) One trocar is inserted on the temporal side. The vitreous cutter is inserted through the trocar and removes the anterior vitreous. (**b**) An irrigation handpiece is held in the anterior chamber

irrigation handpiece is placed in the anterior chamber (Fig. 3.4b). Now an anterior vitrectomy from pars plana is possible. The complete removal of the anterior vitreous is possible.

3.2   Trocar Surgery with Two Trocars

The advantage of two trocars is that the second hand is free (see Video 3.2). The irrigation handpiece is replaced by an infusion line (Fig. 3.5). The infusion line is inserted into one trocar and establishes a stable pressure inside the eye globe

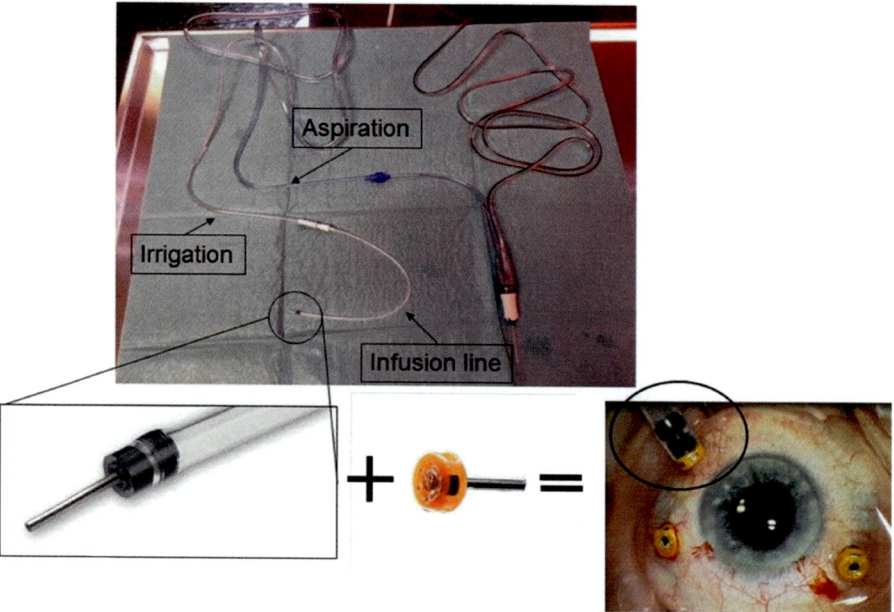

Fig. 3.5 In this setup the irrigation handpiece is replaced by an infusion line. The infusion line is inserted in a trocar. This setup is for *two* or three trocars

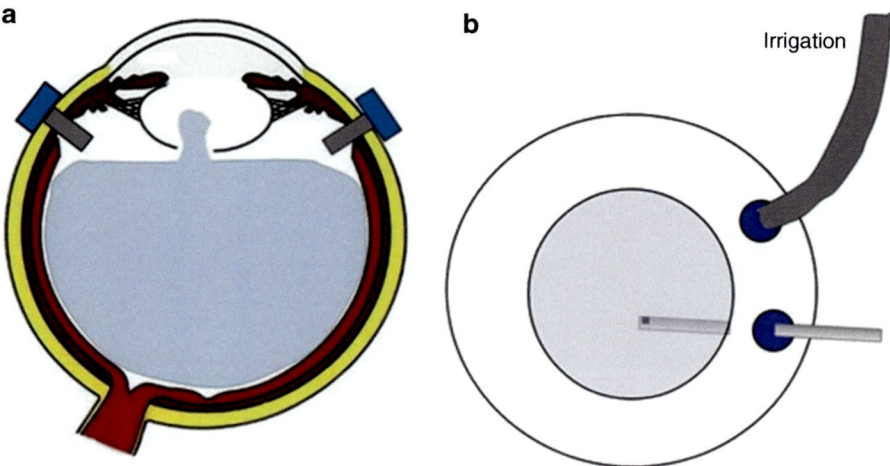

Fig. 3.6 (**a, b**) Trocar surgery with two trocars. One trocar is used for the vitreous cutter and the second trocar is used for the infusion line

(Figs. 3.6 and 3.7). Two trocars are inserted on the temporal side; at 2 and 4 o'clock for the left eye and at 8 and 10 o'clock for the right eye. One trocar is used for the infusion line and the second trocar is used for the vitreous cutter (Fig. 3.4). Alternatively, you can use an anterior chamber maintainer. The disadvantage of an anterior chamber maintainer is that it dislocates easily if you rotate the eye. In contract, a pars plana infusion is stable and does not dislocate. Start trocar surgery with one trocar but move soon over to two trocars. The best trocar surgery technique is with two trocars. The infusion line is placed in the second trocar (Fig. 3.5).

Summary

Start this technique with one trocar cannula. Get acquainted with anterior vitrectomy with one trocar and an irrigation handpiece. Then insert two cannulas and insert an infusion line in the second trocar. Finally get acquainted to perform an anterior vitrectomy with an infusion line (see Fig. 3.8).

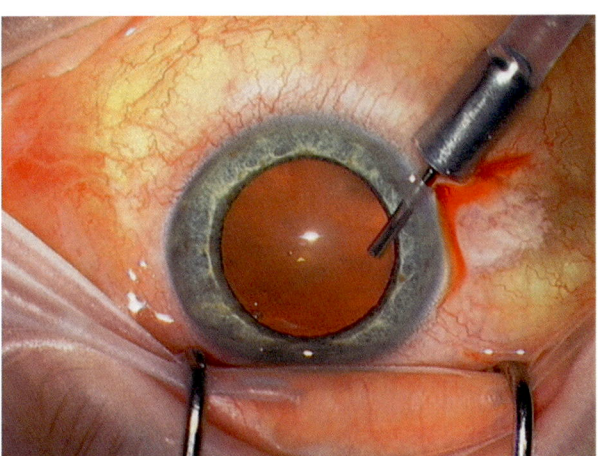

Fig. 3.7 An anterior chamber maintainer is a good alternative to the irrigation handpiece

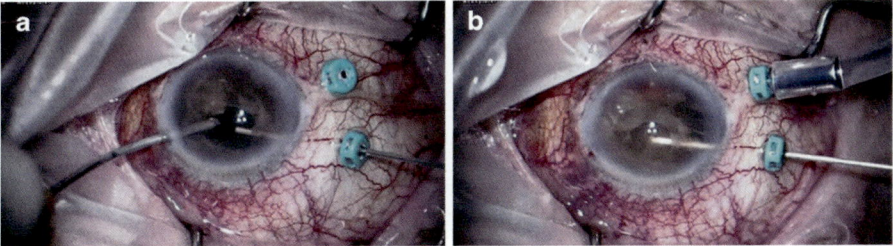

Fig. 3.8 (**a**) Anterior vitrectomy through one trocar with an irrigation handpiece. (**b**) Anterior vitrectomy with two trocars and an infusion line

3.3   Settings for Anterior Vitrectomy on Phacoemulsification Machine

Before operating on a complication on your own, you should have seen this complication managed by an experienced surgeon or in a surgical video. In addition, you have to know exactly the instrumentation and the machine settings for a vitrectomy on a phaco machine. I will therefore add some technical details:

Modern vitreous cutters are *not* coaxial. You need a separate infusion.

The Infinity and Centurion machines (Alcon) offer the following choices for anterior vitrectomy:

1. Cutting-I/A;
2. I/A-cutting;

I recommend the I/A -cutting mode. When you step on the foot pedal slightly, you are in the aspiration mode, when you step firmly on the pedal, you are in the cutting mode. You can cause serious damage during cutting, which is not the case for the I/A mode. It is therefore prudent that a slight stepping on the foot pedal activates I/A (which causes little damage) and a firm stepping on the foot pedal activates vitrectomy (which can cause serious damage).

Settings for Anterior Vitrectomy

If you use two trocars with an infusion line we recommend using continuous irrigation. The globe has a stable IOP and you don't need to worry about irrigation (Fig. 3.9). The irrigation pressure is 45 cmH$_2$O (=33 mmHg) for Infinity machine. Furthermore we recommend Vitrectomy I/A cut. The vitreous cutter has 2500 CPM.

Fig. 3.9 Phaco settings for anterior vitrectomy. We use the same settings for one or two trocars. If you use an irrigation line, then continuous irrigation is activated

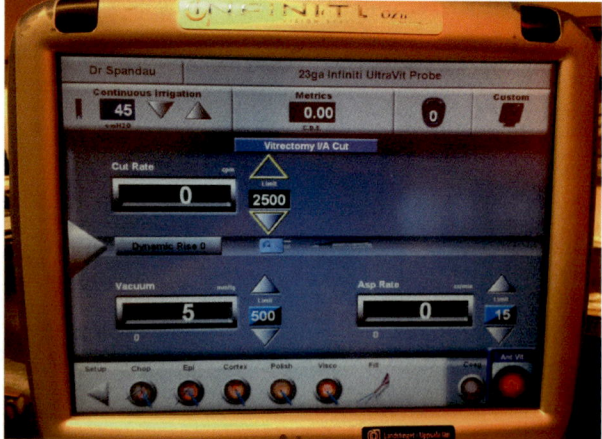

Chapter 4
Basics of Anterior Vitrectomy

4.1 Intraocular Pressure: Clinical Assessment and Surgical Action

The tonus of the globe is an essential element of anterior and especially of posterior segment surgery. As a surgeon you must be able to assess the tonus of the globe and take adequate actions.

Assessment: The intraocular pressure can be assessed in the easiest way with the index finger. During posterior segment surgery you check the globe pressure regularly with your index finger. There are also clinical signs for high and low IOP. If the IOP is too high, then the cornea becomes edematous because the endothelium cannot pump out the excess intracorneal fluid. Further signs are an iris prolapse through the corneal incision and a flat anterior chamber. A low IOP presents with a globe losing its shape, scleral folds occur. In addition, a choroidal detachment develops. In the anterior segment there are hardly signs for a low IOP except for folds in the cornea or a gaping scleral tunnel.

Another important factor is the presence of aphakia or not. If aphakia is present, then intraocular fluid can flow freely from posterior to anterior segment and vice versa. *Remark*: A PCR is more or less comparable to aphakia. In contrast, if a natural lens or in-the-bag IOL is present, then aqueous flows only slowly from posterior to anterior segment and vice versa. For example: In case of aphakia or PCR an anterior chamber maintainer has the same effect as a pars plana trocar infusion because no barrier between anterior and posterior segment is present. If, however, a natural lens or an in-the-bag IOL is present, then an anterior chamber maintainer cannot maintain the IOP in the posterior segment. In case of pseudophakia (or natural lens) you cannot perform an anterior vitrectomy with an anterior chamber maintainer because the fluid flows too slowly from the anterior to the posterior chamber. If you perform in this situation a vitrectomy then an underpressure in the posterior segment will develop. This underpressure may result in a subchoroidal hemorrhage.

© Springer Nature Switzerland AG 2020   25
U. Spandau, *Trocar Surgery for Cataract Surgeons*,
https://doi.org/10.1007/978-3-030-36093-1_4

Surgical procedure: What to do if the IOP is too high? The simplest surgical procedure is a paracentesis. If a paracentesis is not possible because of a flat anterior chamber, then you can relieve pressure from the posterior segment (via pars plana). This can be achieved with a needle cannula or a vitreous cutter. If the IOP is too low, you can increase the IOP by injecting fluid into the anterior chamber or into the posterior chamber (like an intravitreal injection). Assess the effect of your action with the index finger. *Remark*: A normal eye tolerates an intravitreal injection of approximately 0.1 ml fluid without a paracentesis. If you inject 0.2 ml fluid into the vitreous then a paracentesis is required. This is of course not valid for abnormally small eyes.

4.2   Location of Vitreous Prolapse

Vitreous prolapse can be from posterior segment to anterior segment or it can be localized in posterior segment (Fig. 4.2). In either case, it is best removed from pars plana with or without anterior approach. An only anterior approach will remove vitreous inadequately. If the vitreous prolapse is localized anterior to the iris (Fig. 4.1a) then it can only be removed with a vitreous cutter placed anterior to the iris, i.e. from the anterior chamber. If the vitreous prolapse is localized posterior to the iris then the vitreous can be only removed completely from pars plana (Fig. 4.1b). If a vitreous prolapse is present in the anterior chamber, then start with vitrectomy from pars plana (Fig. 4.2a) in order to remove the base of the vitreous prolapse. Then remove the vitreous prolapse from the anterior segment (Fig. 4.2b).

Conventional anterior vitrectomy limbus versus anterior vitrectomy from pars plana.

A conventional anterior vitrectomy is performed from the limbus (Fig. 4.3). The disadvantage of this technique is that it is impossible to perform a complete anterior

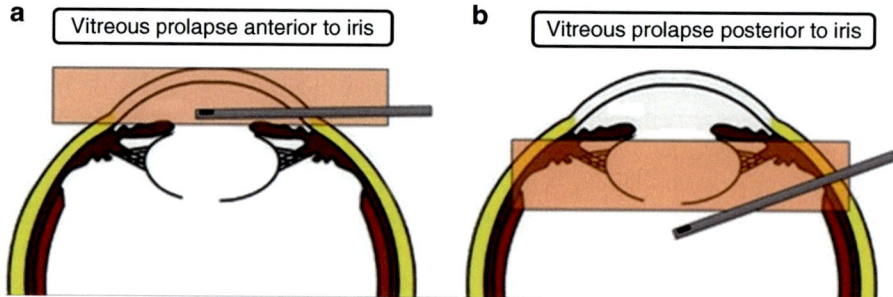

Fig. 4.1 Vitreous prolapse anterior *or* posterior to iris. (**a**) The vitreous prolapse is localized anterior to the iris and is best removed from the anterior segment. (**b**) The vitreous prolapse is localized posterior to the iris and is best removed from pars plana

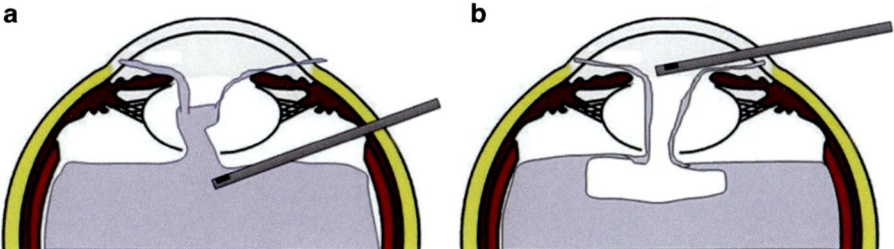

Fig. 4.2 Vitreous prolapse anterior *and* posterior to iris. (**a**) Remove first the anterior vitreous from pars plana. (**b**) Then remove the vitreous strands from the cornea

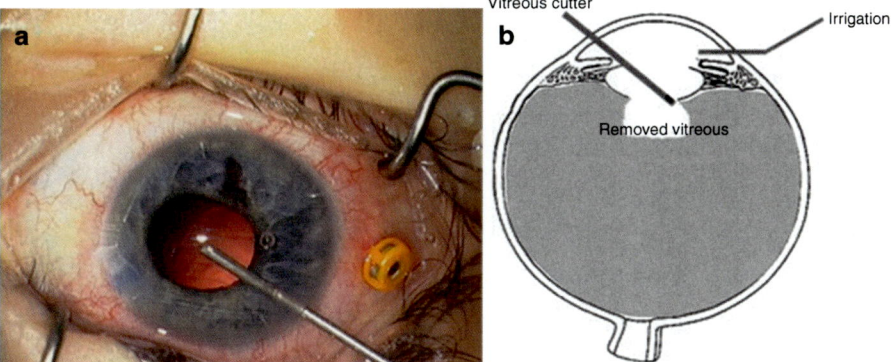

Fig. 4.3 (**a**) An anterior vitrectomy from the limbus. Insert the anterior vitreous cutter through a paracentesis and remove the vitreous prolapse. Caution: Do not forget the infusion (not depicted). (**b**) Drawing of an anterior vitrectomy from the limbus. The disadvantage of this technique is that the anterior vitreous is only inadequately removed. In addition, the lens capsule can be easily damaged

vitrectomy because the iris and the lens capsule are in the way. A conventional anterior vitrectomy results often in a postoperative vitreous prolapse because anterior vitreous is only partially removed.

What is the advantage of an anterior vitrectomy from pars plana compared to a limbal approach? The advantage is that the anterior vitreous is much easier to remove from pars plana, because the iris and the lens capsule are not in the way (Fig. 4.4). In addition, the anterior vitreous can be completely removed from pars plana because the vitreous cutter is located behind the iris and the lens capsule.

An anterior segment surgeon has not much experience with a vitreous cutter. A vitreous cutter is much less powerful than a phacoemulsification handpiece and can, therefore, cause less damage. Which damage can a vitreous cutter cause? If you touch the retina with the vitreous cutter you can damage the retina but that's unlikely. Which is the most common damage with the vitreous cutter? The anterior capsule. Try absolutely to avoid damaging the anterior capsule during anterior vitrectomy.

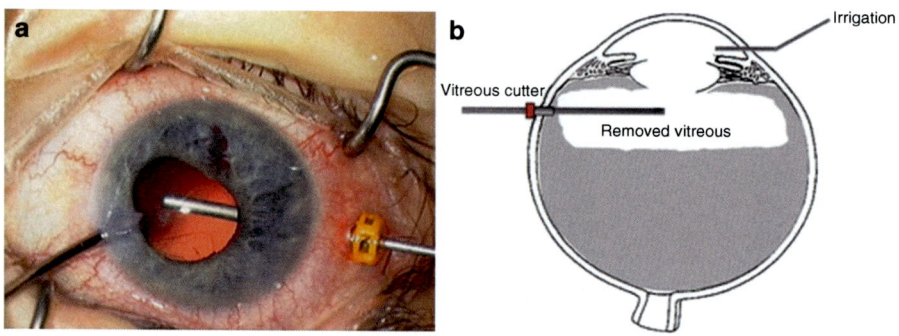

Fig. 4.4 (**a**) An anterior vitrectomy from pars plana. Place the infusion via a paracentesis in the anterior chamber. Then vitrectomize the anterior vitreous from pars plana. (**b**) Drawing of an anterior pars plana vitrectomy from pars plana. Insert a 23G trocar 3.5–4 mm behind the limbus. The advantage of this method is that the anterior vitreous can be completely removed, that the vitrectomy is easier to perform, and a damage of the lens capsule is unlikely

Hold therefore the port of the vitreous cutter away from the lens capsule and point it towards the optic disc. You need an intact anterior capsule to implant a sulcus fixated IOL.

4.3 Dry Versus Wet Vitrectomy

Dry vitrectomy is a vitrectomy without irrigation, wet vitrectomy is with irrigation. Dry vitrectomy is popular amongst elder cataract surgeons because irrigation increases the vitreous prolapse. I want to give here a very strong recommendation to my readers. If you are not an experienced VR surgeon, then use *never* a dry vitrectomy. I have seen many, many terrible complications from dry vitrectomy. What happens, if you do dry vitrectomy? You create an under pressure in the eye, the choroidal vessels rupture and subchoroidal hemorrhage develops with terrible consequences. There is one exception to my recommendation. In positive vitreous pressure you need to do a dry vitrectomy. *Remark*: When you perform a vitrectomy check the IOP with your index finger. If the globe is soft, then stop immediately with vitrectomy.

4.4 Summary

The insertion of a trocar cannula at pars plana increases the surgical spectrum of a cataract surgeon immensely: Anterior vitrectomy from pars plana, the recovery of a dropping nucleus, the elevation of a dislocated IOL in anterior vitreous and removal of a PCO. All these procedures can be performed with a regular phacoemulsification machine.

Chapter 5
Anaesthesia

For cataract surgery we use topical and intracameral anaesthesia and for trocar surgery we use retrobulbar/peribulbar anaesthesia. For the latter we use 50% Carbocain (mepivacain 20 mg/ml) and 50% Marcain (bupivacain 5 mg/ml). Inject 5 cc (ml) inferotemporal through the inferior eyelid.

5.1 Tips and Tricks

If you want to add anaesthetics during an ongoing surgery, then inject 3 ml Carbocain through the caruncle (Fig. 5.1). The caruncle is further away from the sclera which makes it a safe place to inject. In addition, the anaesthetic reaches the retrobulbar space. Wait 1 min before you continue.

Fig. 5.1 Inject 3 ml (cc) Carbocain through the caruncle

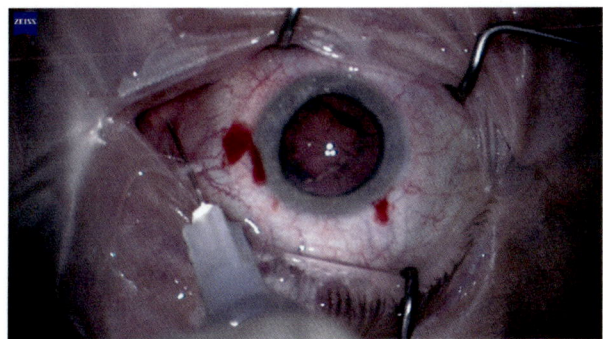

© Springer Nature Switzerland AG 2020
U. Spandau, *Trocar Surgery for Cataract Surgeons*,
https://doi.org/10.1007/978-3-030-36093-1_5

Part III
Trocar Based Surgeries of Anterior Segment

Chapter 6
Check List for Trocar-Based Surgeries of Anterior Segment

Trocar surgery is best learned in a stepwise manner. Start to perform surgeries with one trocar and proceed later on with two trocars. The following checklist may be a guide for your surgical development:

How to Learn Trocar Surgery for an Anterior Segment Surgeon in a Stepwise Manner. See the Following Check List

1. Insertion and removal of one trocar on the temporal side.
2. Anterior vitrectomy through trocar cannula.
3. Master SICS.
4. Elevation of anterior dislocated nucleus.
5. Elevation of anterior dislocated IOL.
6. Secondary IOL implantation.
7. Insertion of two trocars on the temporal side. One trocar for irrigation line.
8. Anterior vitrectomy from pars plana with infusion line.

Start trocar surgery with steps 1–2 and get acquainted to this new technique. The next steps require that you master SICS (step 3). Then try to elevate a subluxated nucleus, extract it through a scleral tunnel and then continue with an anterior vitrectomy through trocar cannulas (step 4). Similarly, you can elevate and extract an anterior dislocated IOL and perform a secondary IOL implantation (steps 5–6). The next big step is the insertion of two trocar cannulas. The second trocar cannula is used for the infusion (=irrigation line). The irrigation line gives you two free hands. Perform an anterior vitrectomy and all other surgeries with two trocars (steps 7–8). It is important to get acquainted to two trocars before you proceed to posterior segment procedures.

© Springer Nature Switzerland AG 2020
U. Spandau, *Trocar Surgery for Cataract Surgeons*,
https://doi.org/10.1007/978-3-030-36093-1_6

Chapter 7
The Surgical Technique of Insertion of Trocar Cannulas

The insertion of trocar cannulas is technically easy and fast to learn. It is similar to an intravitreal injection. See one, do one.

7.1 Anatomy of Pars Plana

The trocar cannulas are placed in the pars plana. Pars plana is a landmark in the ocular wall but the surgery is done in the vitreous. The pars plana is located between the ciliary body and the retina and devoid of retina (Fig. 7.1). This feature makes the pars plana an excellent place for insertion of trocars or instruments into the posterior cavity.

Two Types of Sclerotomy
There are two types of sclerotomy (Fig. 7.2). The first (traditional) sclerotomy is performed perpendicular. Open the conjunctiva and perform a perpendicular sclerotomy (ideally with a V-lance from Alcon). This sclerotomy is 20G big and is

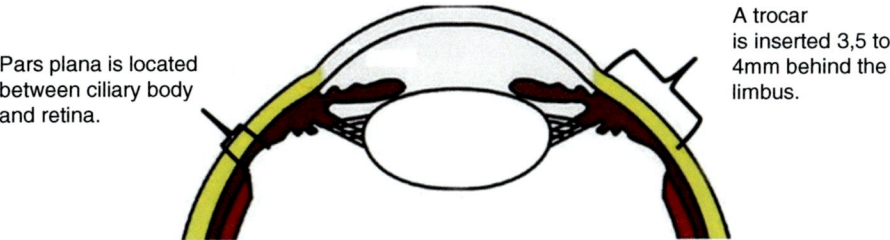

Pars plana is located between ciliary body and retina.

A trocar is inserted 3,5 to 4mm behind the limbus.

Fig. 7.1 The pars plana is located between ciliary body and retina. The retina is absent at the pars plana region. This feature makes the pars plana the perfect anatomic place for insertion of instruments into the posterior segment of the eye

© Springer Nature Switzerland AG 2020
U. Spandau, *Trocar Surgery for Cataract Surgeons*,
https://doi.org/10.1007/978-3-030-36093-1_7

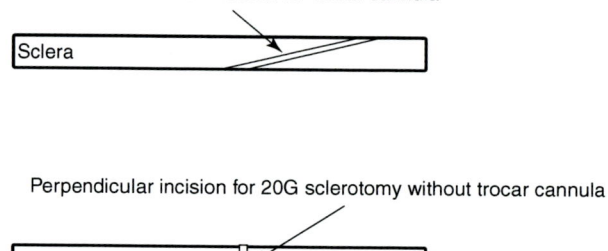

Fig. 7.2 There are two types of sclerotomy. In case of a trocar cannula the sclerotomy is lamellar resulting in a watertight closure of the sclerotomy. In case of a 20G sclerotomy without trocar cannula a perpendicular incision is made. This sclerotomy is not watertight and has to be consequently sutured

Fig. 7.3 20G sclerotomy with a 20G V lance from Alcon

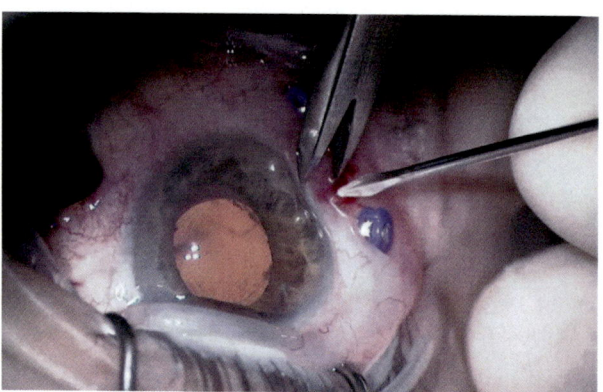

used for fragmatome. No trocar cannula is inserted in this sclerotomy. This sclerotomy is not watertight and requires a suture, ideally a X-stitch. The second (new) sclerotomy is lamellar. A trocar is inserted in a 15 deg. angle through conjunctiva and sclera. A trocar cannula is left in this 23G sclerotomy. This lamellar sclerotomy is watertight after removal of the trocar cannula. A suture is usually not required.

7.2 20G Sclerotomy Without Trocar Cannulas

Instruments: 20G V lance (Alcon)
Open the conjunctiva focally. Mark the sclera with a scleral marker or a caliper. Introduce the knife (the blade is parallel to the limbus) straight towards the center of the eye (Fig. 7.3). At the end of the surgery exclude and remove a possible vitreous prolapse and close the sclerotomy with a Vicryl 8–0 cross suture. Then close the conjunctiva with a Vicryl 8–0 suture.

7.3   23G Sclerotomy with Trocar Cannulas

7.3.1   Instruments: Trocars (Mani, FCI, DORC, Aurolab)

1. Mark the sclerotomy.
2. Insertion of the trocar.

Insert a trocar at 3 or 9 o'clock. Measure and mark the sclerotomy with a scleral marker (Fig. 7.4a), a caliper or with the trocar 3.5–4 mm posterior to the limbus. It

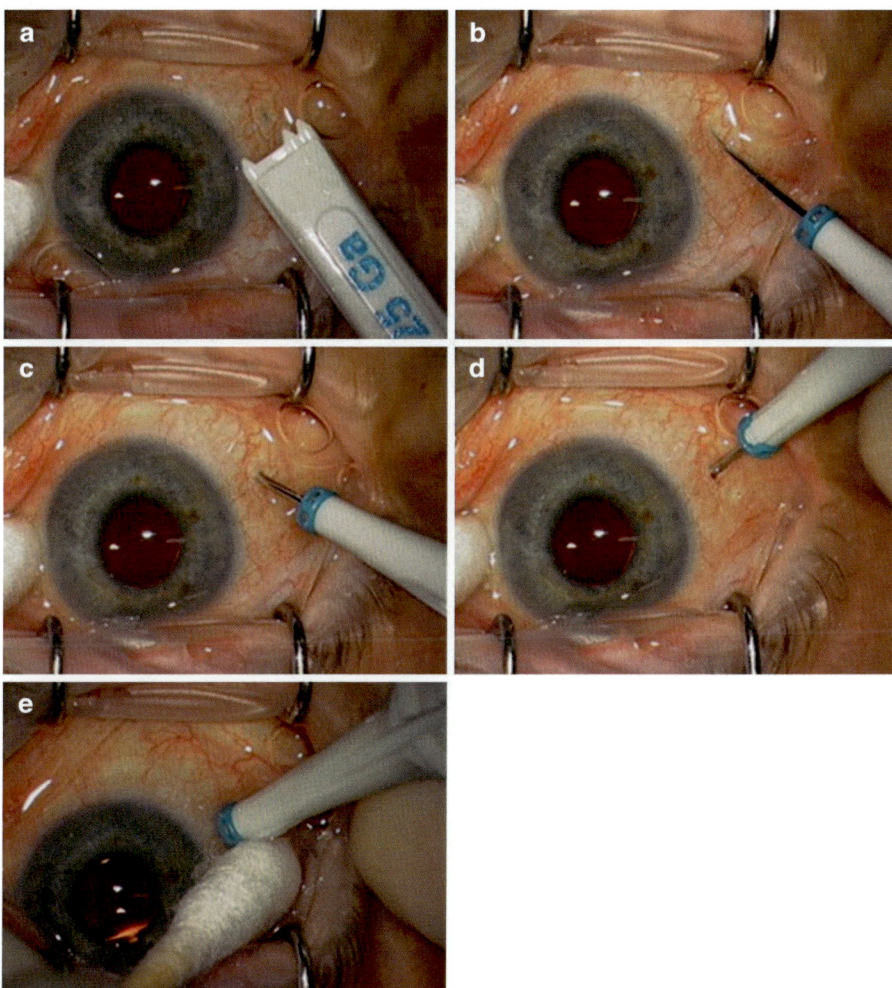

Fig. 7.4 Insertion of a trocar: (**a**) Fixate the globe with a cotton swab. Mark the sclerotomy with the trocar marker (3.5–4 mm). (**b**) Insert the trocar in an angle of 15–20° through the conjunctiva and sclera. (**c, d**) Then insert the second half in direction of the middle of the eye. (**e**) Fixate the cannula with a forceps and remove the handpiece. The trocar cannula remains in the sclera

is advisable to fixate the eyeball simultaneously with forceps or a cotton wool swab. Insert the knife in an angle of 15° to the limbus and stab the knife through the conjunctiva and the sclera (Fig. 7.4a). If you are half way through (Fig. 7.4c), raise the inserter and stab the knife for the second half in direction of the middle of the eye (perpendicular) (Fig. 7.4d, e). Then fixate the trocar with a cannula holding forceps or an anatomic forceps or cotton swab and pull out the trocar handpiece (Fig. 7.4e).

Removal of Trocar

Remove the trocar cannula with a trocar forceps (DORC) or an anatomical forceps. Then press the tip of the forceps against the sclera so that the wedges of the sclerotomy get attached to each other. A suture is usually not required. In case of a suture close the sclerotomy with a Vicryl 8-0 suture.

Tips and Tricks

Insertion of trocars: The insertion of a trocar is almost identical to an intravitreal injection. The only difference is that an injection is performed completely perpendicular (to the middle of the eye) whereas the trocar is inserted for the first half lamellar and the second half perpendicular.

Chapter 8
The Surgical Technique of Anterior Vitrectomy from Pars Plana

The anterior vitrectomy from pars plana with trocar cannulas is easy to learn. The insertion of trocars is simple, and the advantages will become immediately obvious.

The Video 2.1 demonstrates the basics and the setup of a vitreous cutter.

Instruments
1. 23G trocar
2. 23G vitreous cutter

Individual Steps
1. Insertion of trocar
2. Anterior vitrectomy from pars plana
3. Removal of trocar

The Surgery Step-by Step
1. Insertion of trocar

    The major step for a cataract surgeon regarding this technique is the insertion of a trocar cannula. But this is really simple and easy to learn. And it requires no suture. Insert one 23G trocar 3,5 mm behind the limbus at 9 o'clock (right eye) or 3 o'clock (left eye).
2. Anterior vitrectomy from pars plana

    Instrumentation:
    - Non-dominant hand: Irrigation handpiece
    - Dominant hand: Vitreous cutter

Normally the anterior vitrectomy is carried out bimanually (like I/A). The vitreous cutter removes tissue and fluid and an irrigation handpiece provides irrigation fluid, in order to avoid a hypotension. Begin by placing the irrigation cannula in the anterior chamber. Then insert the vitreous cutter in the trocar until you can view the

© Springer Nature Switzerland AG 2020
U. Spandau, *Trocar Surgery for Cataract Surgeons*,
https://doi.org/10.1007/978-3-030-36093-1_8

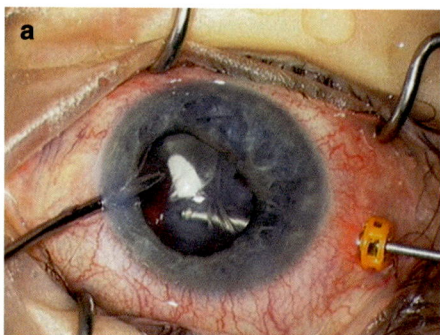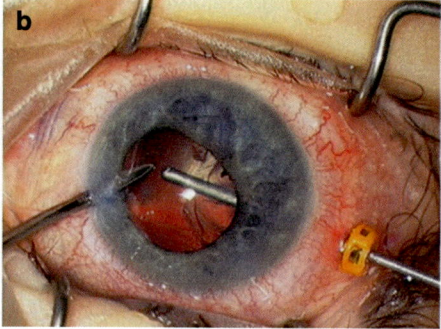

Fig. 8.1 (**a**) The irrigation handpiece is inserted through the paracentesis. The vitreous cutter is inserted through the trocar. Remove first the cortex from pars plana. Caution: Use only aspiration and NO cutting. (**b**) Then continue with removal of the vitreous prolapse. Hold the opening of the vitreous cutter towards the posterior pole. Make circular movements along the edge of the pupil. Continue with these slow circular movements for approximately 5 min. Then you have removed sufficient anterior vitreous

tip behind the pupil. Turn the port of the vitreous cutter towards the optic disc and cut the anterior vitreous. Make circular movements along the edge of the pupil and stay at the same horizontal level (Fig. 8.1). This manoeuvre takes approximately 5 min. You can also turn the port of the vitreous cutter sideways but not upwards, because you can easily damage the capsule. If you are unsure, if residual vitreous is present in the anterior chamber, then inject triamcinolone into the anterior chamber to stain the vitreous.

Tips and Tricks

When there is vitreous in anterior chamber with remnant cortex, it is better to do vitrectomy first. If you want to remove the cortex first by aspiration, there is a high chance that you pull on the entangled vitreous leading to traction on retina. If you are experienced with the vitreous cutter, then I recommend using the vitreous cutter for vitreous removal *and* cortex removal. If you remove the vitreous, you work with cutting function and if you remove the cortex, you work with aspiration function. Start with anterior vitrectomy from the pars plana to cut all attachment of vitreous from behind. Then aspirate the cortex and if necessary cut residual vitreous. All procedure done with a cutter alone so that you can alter between cutting and aspiration with footswitch, if needed. But you must be cautious not to injure the lens capsule with the vitreous cutter.

3. Removal of Trocar

    Remove the trocar with anatomical forceps (Fig. 8.2a). Then press on the sclerotomy with anatomic forceps to avoid leaking (Fig. 8.2b). Check for vitreous strand in the sclerotomy and remove it in case with the vitreous cutter. If the sclerotomy is leaking, then suture it with a Vicryl 8-0 interrupted stitch.

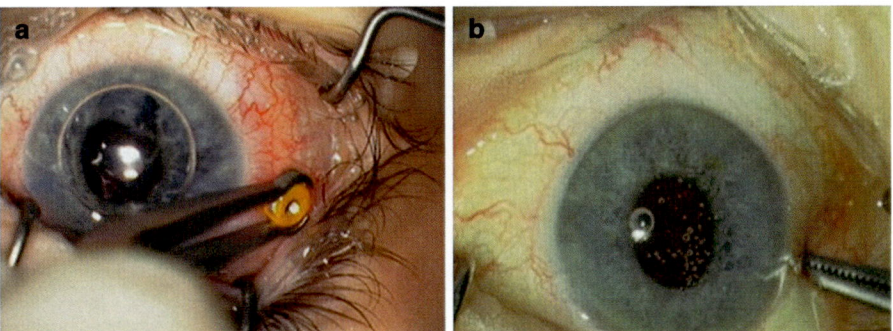

Fig. 8.2 (**a**) Remove the trocar with a trocar forceps (DORC) or anatomic forceps. (**b**) Then close the sclerotomy by pressing against it with anatomic forceps

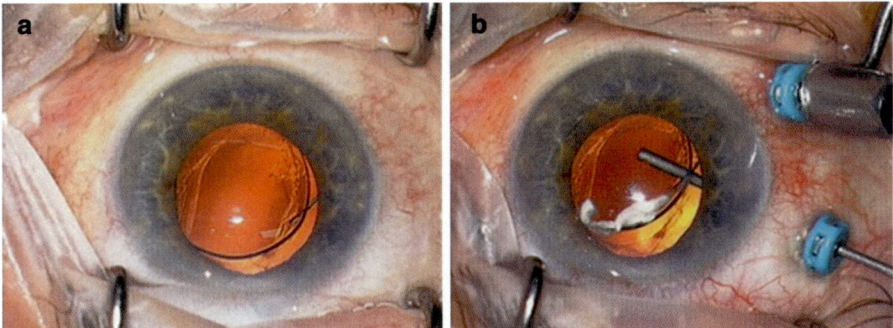

Fig. 8.3 (**a**) A vitreous prolapse after posterior capsular defect. The vitreous prolapse is difficult to detect under the operation microscope. (**b**) After staining with triamcinolone, the vitreous prolapse is easy to detect

Tips and Tricks
Staining of the vitreous prolapse with triamcinolone: Volon A, Kenalog, Squibb: Indication: staining of the vitreous after a posterior capsule rupture (Fig. 8.3). Dilute triamcinolone 1:3 with BSS (3 ml BSS and 1 ml triamcinolone). Inject a volume of approximately 0,2 cc diluted triamcinolone into the anterior chamber and after a few seconds wash it out with BSS.

Tips and Tricks
Low IOP: (1) Inject BSS through a side port. (2) Inject BSS with a cannula through the trocar cannula into the posterior segment until IOP is normal. (3) If no trocar cannula is present: Inject BSS with a 30G cannula into the posterior segment until the IOP is normal.

Chapter 9
Surgical Management of Dislocated Cortical Fragments

Cortical or nuclear fragments may dislocate behind the lens capsule into the so-called Berger space (Fig. 9.1). The Berger space is the space between the patellar fossa of the vitreous and the lens. In case of a zonular defect cortical fragments may dislocate through the zonular defect into the Berger space (Figs. 9.1 and 9.2). A removal from the anterior chamber is not possible. The only possibility to remove a cortical fragment at this location is from pars plana.

The Video 9.1 demonstrates the surgical management of dislocated cortical fragments.

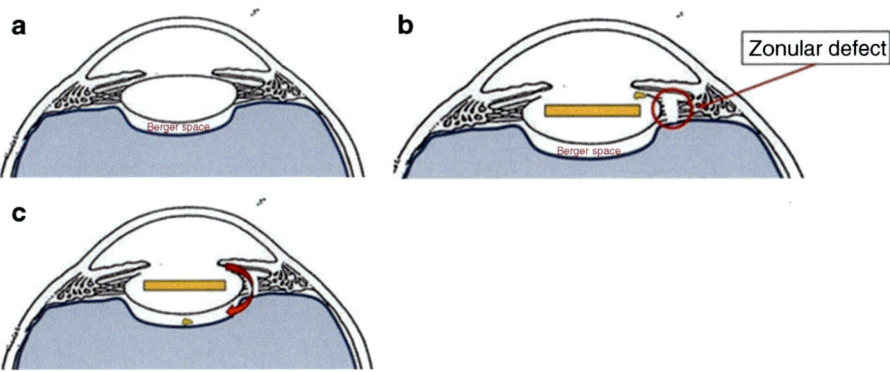

Fig. 9.1 (**a**) The Berger space is the space between the anterior hyaloid and the lens. (**b**) A cortical or nuclear fragment may dislocate through a zonular defect into the Berger space. (**c**) The lens capsule is intact. It is impossible to remove the fragment from the anterior chamber; it can only be removed from pars plana

Electronic Supplementary Material The online version of this chapter (https://doi.org/10.1007/978-3-030-36093-1_9) contains supplementary material, which is available to authorized users.

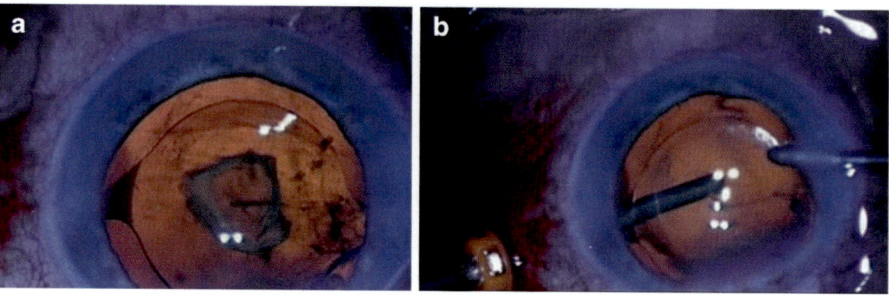

Fig. 9.2 (**a**) A cortical fragment is located behind the intact lens capsule. (**b**) A trocar cannula is inserted on the temporal side. The cortical fragment is removed with a 23G anterior vitreous cutter (Alcon)

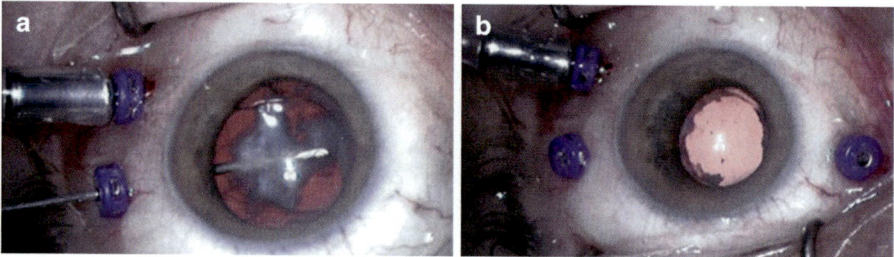

Fig. 9.3 (**a**) Cortical material is located behind the IOL. A posterior capsular rupture is present and the IOL is located in the sulcus. (**b**) Insert one or two trocars and remove the cortical material from pars plana. If cortical material drops then you insert three trocar cannulas in order to remove the dropped cortex from the posterior cavity

Surgical Technique

Instruments
1. One or two 23G trocars
2. One anterior vitreous cutter

The Surgery in Detail
Insert one or two trocars at the temporal side. Place the tip of the vitreous cutter behind the cortical fragment and cut cautiously in order not to injure the lens capsule (Fig. 9.2).

It may happen that a posterior capsular rupture occurs when cortical material is still present in the eye. The surgeon implants the IOL in the sulcus. The cortical material is located behind the IOL. Then he refers the patient for removal of cortical fragments. You can try to remove the cortical material with I/A from corneal incision but the vitreous prolapse makes cortex removal difficult. The best technique is, therefore, the removal from pars plana (Fig. 9.3). Insert one or two trocars on the temporal side. Place the tip of the cutter behind the cortical fragments. It may happen that the cortical material drops through the capsular rupture. In this case be prepared to continue vitrectomy with three trocars, viewing system and light fiber.

Remark In case of a PCR when cortical or nuclear fragments are present it is advisable to place the IOL *behind* the fragments to prevent a drop through the capsular rupture (IOL scaffold).

Chapter 10
Surgical Management of Posterior Capsular Opacification from Pars Plana

In children or handicapped patients, a YAG capsulotomy cannot be performed. An alternative is a capsulectomy from pars plana.

The Video 10.1 demonstrates the surgical management of posterior capsular opacification from pars plana.

Vitrector Settings
200 cuts per min, normal vacuum

Surgical Technique of Removal of PCO from Pars Plana
Insert one or two trocars 3.5 mm behind the limbus at 3 o'clock (LE) or 9 o'clock (RE). Perform round circular movements with the vitreous cutter until a central and round opening is present (Fig. 10.1). An anterior vitrectomy is not necessary.

Postoperative Treatment
Combined Dexamethasone-Gentamicin drops 3x daily for 3 weeks. Mydriatics are not necessary.

Electronic Supplementary Material The online version of this chapter (https://doi.org/10.1007/978-3-030-36093-1_10) contains supplementary material, which is available to authorized users.

U. Spandau, *Trocar Surgery for Cataract Surgeons*,
https://doi.org/10.1007/978-3-030-36093-1_10

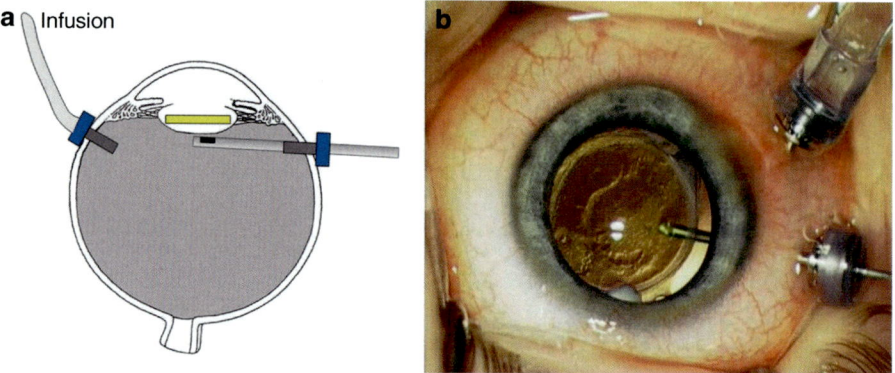

Fig. 10.1   (**a**) A thick PCO is present. (**b**) Removal of posterior capsular opacification from pars plana

Chapter 11
Surgical Management of Positive Vitreous Pressure (PVP) During Cataract Surgery

The Video 11.1 demonstrates the surgical management of positive vitreous pressure (PVP).

When the anterior chamber becomes shallow during phacoemulsification, the surgeon must promptly evaluate its potential cause. A decisive determinant in the differential diagnosis is the hardness of the globe, which the surgeon must palpate. Firmness signals positive vitreous pressure (PVP); softness indicates its absence. PVP is a phenomenon characterized by forward displacement of the lens-iris diaphragm during phacoemulsification that can lead to a cascade of intraoperative complications, potentially with devastating results. Cataract surgeons need to understand the causes of a shallow anterior chamber [1, 2]. See Video 11.1.

Pathomechanism of PVP is an aqueous misdirection; the misdirection of BSS behind the lens capsule or behind the nucleus. The latter case, misdirection of BSS behind the nucleus, occurs commonly during hydrodissection. The typical cascade of surgical mistakes goes like this: An inexperienced surgeon performs a too small rhexis. Then he/she continues with hydrodissection. There is no effect because the nucleus cannot move due to the small rhexis. Now comes the mistake: The inexperienced surgeon injects additional BSS into the lens capsule. The BSS inflates the lens capsule (Fig. 11.1a) and pushes the nucleus towards the iris creating a pupillary block. This leads to an angle closure as the lens and iris shift forward, exacerbating the elevation of IOP (Fig. 11.1b).

In the past, surgeons used 3 ml or even 5 ml syringes for hydro procedures leading to tremendous amount of vitreous hydration in case of a posterior capsular rupture. A particular mention is for small pupil cases where the surgeons blindly do a hydroprocedure and inadvertently inject fluid over the CCC behind the lens capsule.

Electronic Supplementary Material The online version of this chapter (https://doi. org/10.1007/978-3-030-36093-1_11) contains supplementary material, which is available to authorized users.

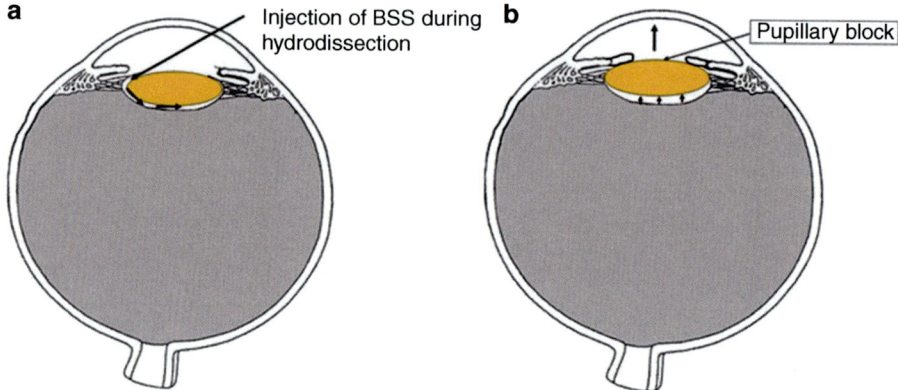

Fig. 11.1 (**a**) A beginner cataract surgeon performs a small capsular rhexis. During hydrodissection he/she injects a high volume of BSS into the lens capsule. The BSS cannot escape due to the too small rhexis. (**b**) The lens capsule is inflated and creates a ciliary block and pupillary block. The iris-lens diaphragma is pushed forwards resulting in a shallow anterior chamber

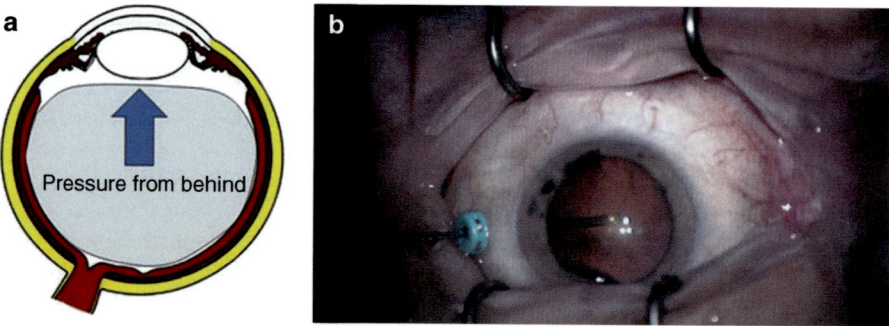

Fig. 11.2 (**a**) Positive vitreous pressure during cataract surgery. (**b**) Perform an anterior vitrectomy from pars plana to relieve pressure. Note that there is no infusion

This fluid can go through the zonules into the vitreous cavity leading to a PVP due to vitreous hydration particularly if you inject copious amount. A PVP, however, may also occur during IOL implantation. There is no explanation available in the literature. The patient can strain and squeeze eyelids resulting in PVP, or if having cough thereby increasing intrathoracic pressure and causing PVP.

Surgical Treatment of PVP
The anterior chamber is shallow, and the iris prolapses through the incisions. Remove slowly all instruments. Now you can do three things: (1) Wait approximately 15–20 min. The intraocular fluid will slowly resorb, the IOP will decrease and you can try to continue surgery. (2) Stop surgery. Give the patient two acetazolamide tablets and continue surgery a few hours later. (3) Perform a dry anterior vitrectomy (Fig. 11.2). Dry vitrectomy means a vitrectomy without irrigation. You

perform a short core vitrectomy until the pressure of the globe has normalized. It is very important to perform only a short vitrectomy. *Remark*: If you remove too much vitreous resulting in an under pressure, then a suprachoroidal hemorrhage may develop.

Surgery of Dry Vitrectomy
Insert one trocar on the temporal side. An irrigation is not required because it will increase the IOP even more. Then place the vitreous cutter behind the nucleus, hold it stable and perform vitrectomy. The opening of the vitreous cutter is pointed towards the optic disc. During vitrectomy place your finger tip on the limbus to feel the pressure of the globe. In the beginning of the procedure the globe is hard but after a few seconds the globe becomes soft. If the globe has approximately an IOP of 10 mmHg stop with vitrectomy. Inflate the anterior chamber with BSS and continue surgery.

Tips and Tricks (Fig. 11.3)
A vitreous decompression can also be performed with a needle cannula. Attach a 23G or 25G needle cannula to a 3 cc syringe. Insert the cannula 3.5 mm behind the limbus and push the cannula forward until the tip of the needle is located in the middle of the eye. Then aspirate 0.2–0.3 ml of fluid. Inflate next the anterior chamber with BSS and continue with cataract surgery.

Remark The technique may cause vitreous traction. It should therefore only be performed in old patients. In this age group the PVD is usually complete and the vitreous is sufficiently liquefied. In contrast, this technique may fail in young eyes because the vitreous is intact and no fluid can be extracted.

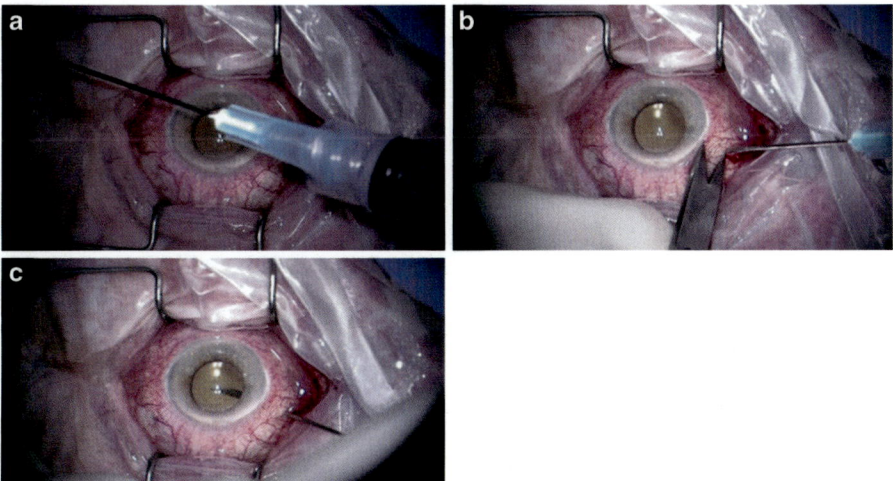

Fig. 11.3 (**a**) Attach a 23G or 25G needle cannula to a 3 cc syringe. (**b**) Insert the needle 3.5 mm behind the limbus. (**c**) Extract fluid from vitreous cavity

References

1. Fishkind WJ. Positive pressure. J Cataract Refract Surg. Pages 95–100; 2009.
2. Chronopoulos A, Thumann G, Schutz J. Positive vitreous pressure: pathophysiology, complications, prevention, and management. Surv Ophthalmol. 2017;62:127e133.

Chapter 12
Surgical Management of a Dropping Nucleus

A dropped nucleus is the most dreaded complication of a cataract surgeon. If you learn this surgical technique, then you can manage the vast majority of dropped nucleus cases on your own.

This technique requires swift action. As soon as you observe a posterior capsular rent, and/or a dropping nucleus then stop phacoemulsification. If the nucleus remains stable, then insert a trocar cannula. Then insert the viscoelastic cannula through the trocar cannula, inject viscoelastics behind the nucleus and then elevate the nucleus into the anterior chamber. *Remark:* The maneuver is easier, if you straighten the angled viscoelastic canula.

Remark: If you have no time to insert a trocar cannula, then attach a 27G needle cannula to the viscoelastic syringe, pierce the sclera—like an intravitreal injection—and inject viscoelastics (Viscoat®) behind the nucleus. Then lift the nucleus into the anterior chamber (Fig. 12.1).

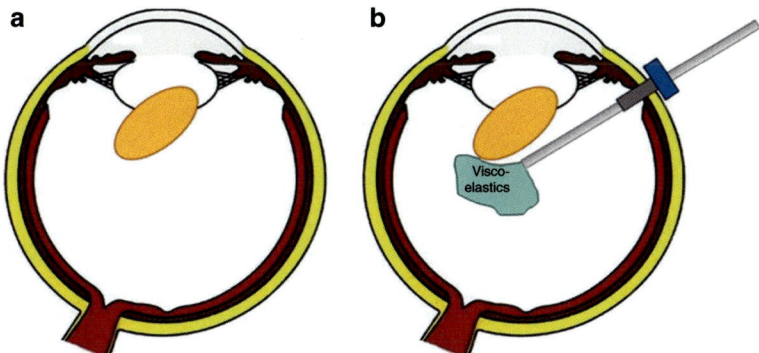

Fig. 12.1 *Dropping nucleus.* (**a**) A subluxated nucleus is difficult to elevate from the limbus because you have to access the nucleus from the back. (**b**) The nucleus is easy to reach from pars plana. Insert a trocar, inject viscoelastics behind the nucleus and elevate it forward inside the anterior chamber (viscolevitation)

© Springer Nature Switzerland AG 2020
U. Spandau, *Trocar Surgery for Cataract Surgeons*,
https://doi.org/10.1007/978-3-030-36093-1_12

Chapter 13
Surgical Management of a Posterior Capsular Rent (PCR)

A posterior capsular rent (PCR) creates a major disturbance in the OR (Fig. 13.1). The calm surgeon becomes agitated and the experienced scrub nurse nervous. Why? Because a PCR is a rare event resulting in an erratic management of a PCR.

The Videos 13.1, 13.2, 13.3, 13.4, 13.5, 13.6, and 13.7 demonstrate the surgical management of a posterior capsular rent (PCR):

In the following, the surgical management will be explained in a clear and simple way. We propose a surgical technique with usage of trocars. One or two trocars are required for the subsequent surgical procedure.

The subsequent surgical procedure depends on during which step of phacoemulsification the posterior capsule was ruptured. If the posterior capsule ruptured during phacoemulsification, then nuclear fragments remain and have to be removed first. See the treatment algorithm Fig. 13.2. If you continue with phacoemulsification the nuclear fragments will drop through the capsular rupture into the vitreous cavity. You can prevent this to happen by first injecting viscoelastic behind the posterior capsule defect. The next step is to remove the lens fragments manually. Elevate the fragments into the anterior chamber and place them on the iris. Then you have to widen the main incision according to the size of the nuclear fragment. See the treatment algorithm Fig. 13.3. An extraction of a big nucleus fragment ($\geq$ ¾ nucleus) via cornea is not advisable because a very large corneal incision and many sutures are needed. A high postoperative astigmatism will be the result. The optimal surgical technique for extraction of a big nucleus fragment is the SICS technique. This technique is described in detail in a later chapter of this book. The fragments can then be removed with the fragment forceps or viscoelastics (Viscoat®). If the posterior capsule ruptured during I/A, then only the residual cortex has to be removed.

Electronic Supplementary Material The online version of this chapter (https://doi.org/10.1007/978-3-030-36093-1_13) contains supplementary material, which is available to authorized users.

Fig. 13.1 Vitreous
prolapse secondary to
posterior capsular rent

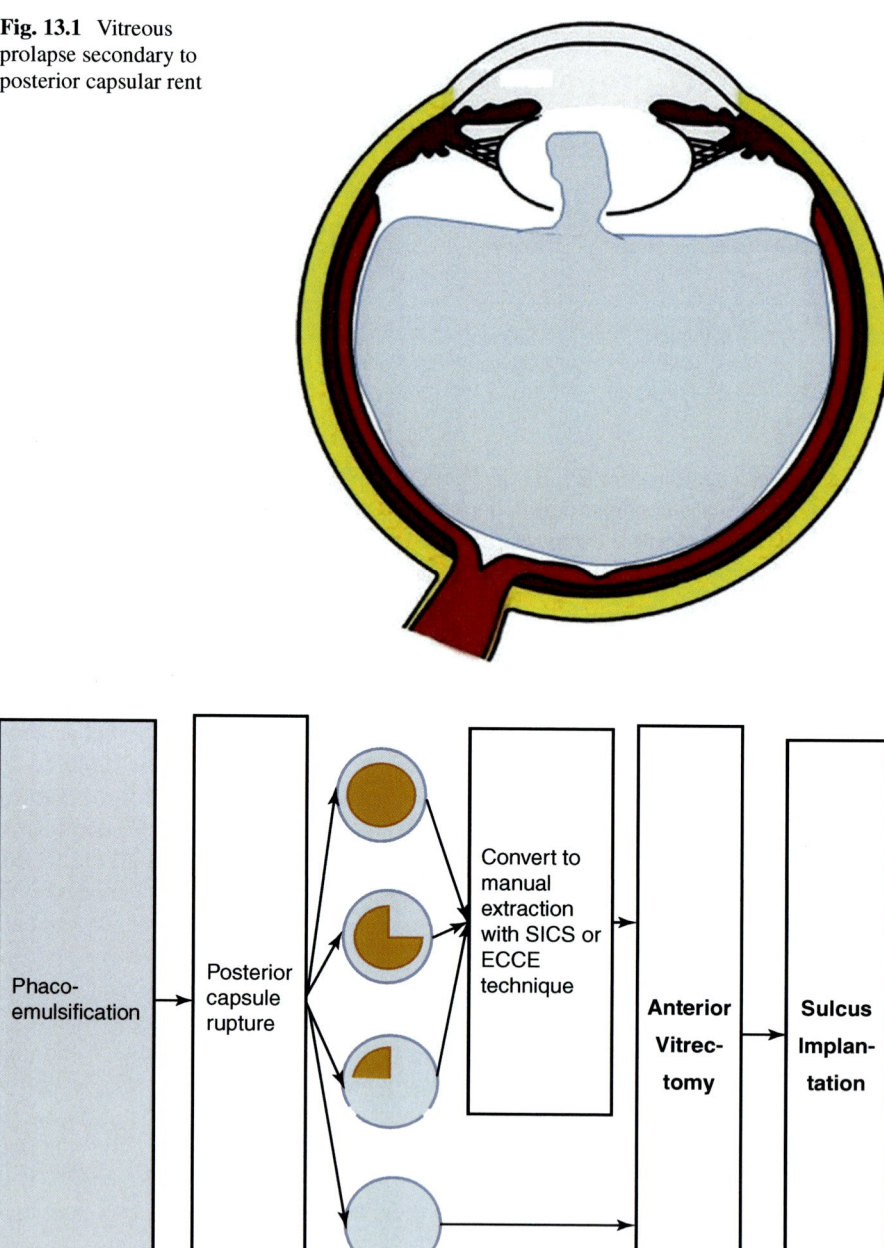

Fig. 13.2 Our treatment algorithm for a posterior capsular rent. Depending on the timing of the capsular defect and the size of the nucleus different techniques are recommended. If nucleus remains when PCR occurs, then remove this fragment manually. Do not use phacoemulsification, the fragment will drop. If *no* nucleus remains, then you can continue immediately with anterior vitrectomy

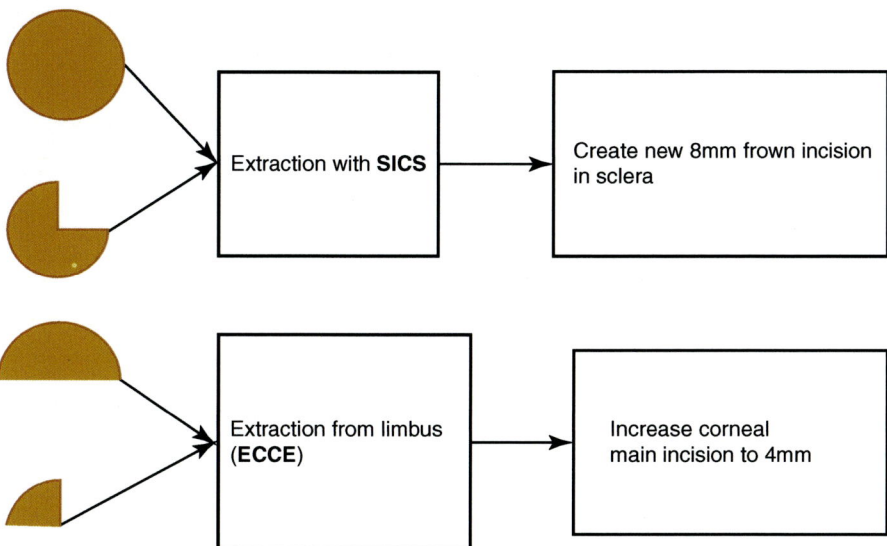

Fig. 13.3 Depending on the size of the nucleus the extraction is performed from the old main incision or a new scleral incision

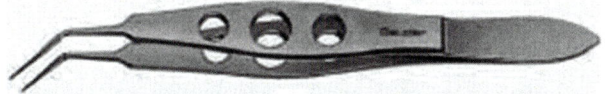

Fig. 13.4 A fragment removal forceps after Gaskin. Indication: Removal of nuclear fragments during a complicated cataract surgery. Geuder, 31,624

Instruments
1. Fragment forceps (Fig. 13.4)
2. Vitreous cutter for phaco machine
3. Trocar

Dye
Triamcinolone (Fig. 13.5)

Individual Steps
1. Viscoelastics into the lens capsule
2. Insertion of 1–2 trocars
3. Luxation of lens fragments into the anterior chamber
4. Widen main incision
5. Extraction of nuclear fragments
6. Injection of triamcinolone into the anterior chamber
7. Anterior vitrectomy and removal of cortex

Fig. 13.5 Kenalog®
(Triamcinolone) stains the
vitreous well. Dilute
triamcinolone with BSS
(1:3). Inject approximately
0.2 ml into the anterior
chamber and wash it after
a few seconds out with
BSS

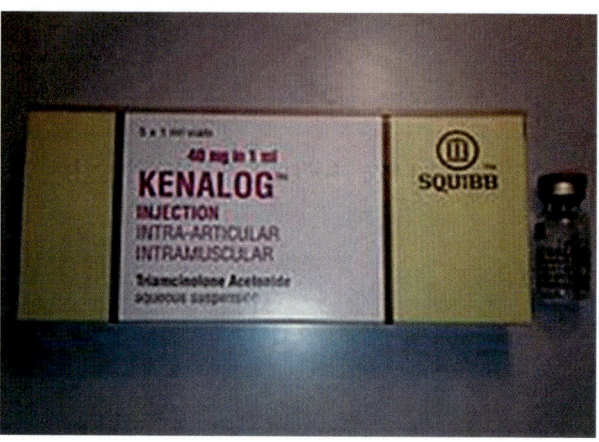

8. Removal of vitreous strand
9. Insert iris hooks
10. IOL implantation in the sulcus
11. Trocar removal

The Surgery Step-by-Step
1. Viscoelastics into the lens capsule
2. Insertion of 1–2 trocars
3. Luxation of lens fragments into the anterior chamber

Inject viscoelastics (Viscoat®) into the capsular bag, so that the vitreous prolapse is pushed back (Fig. 13.6). If the eye is not vitrectomized then the vitreous together with the viscoelastics will be a barrier for the nuclear fragments. If nucleus fragments are still present in the capsular bag, elevate the nuclear fragments with a nucleus manipulator onto the iris (Fig. 13.6). Then insert one or two trocars on the temporal side. It is a common mistake to continue with phacoemulsification after a posterior capsular rent with remaining nucleus. The risk that the nuclear fragment will drop into the vitreous cavity is very high. Remove, therefore, the nucleus manually.

Tips and Tricks
PCR: If a PCR occurs during I/A then remove the aspiration handpiece but leave the irrigation handpiece in the anterior chamber. Then inject Viscoat® into the lens capsule under irrigation. Finally, remove the irrigation handpiece. Similarly, if PCR happens during phacoemulsification, remain in irrigation mode (footswitch position 1). Do not take out the phaco handpiece outside the AC. Inject Viscoat through sideport and fill the AC. Then remove the phaco handpiece.

4. Widen main incision
5. Extraction of nuclear fragments

Continue with widening of the main incision according to the size of the nuclear fragment. See treatment algorithm Fig. 13.7. If 75%–100% of the nucleus has to be

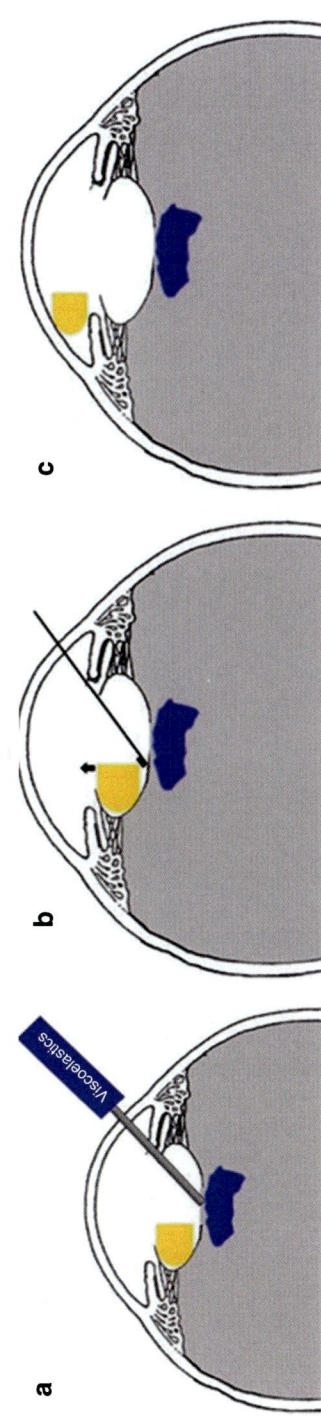

Fig. 13.6 (**a**) If you detect a posterior capsular defect inject first viscoelastics (Viscoat®) to push the vitreous prolapse back and to stabilize the lens capsule with the nucleus. (**b**) Then lift the nuclear fragments up with a nucleus manipulator and place them on the iris. (**c**) The nuclear fragments are safe on the iris. Then widen the main incision and remove the nuclear fragments

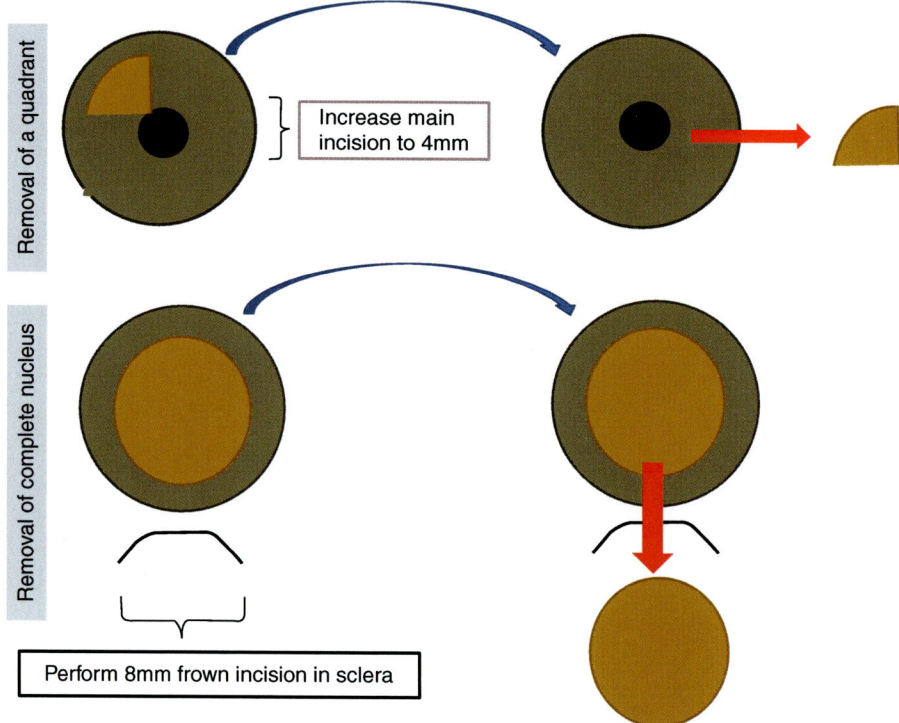

Fig. 13.7 The next step is the manual extraction of the nuclear fragments. Small nuclear fragments can be removed from a widened main incision. Large nuclear fragments should be removed from a large scleral frown incision

extracted, then perform an 8 mm wide frown incision in the sclera. If 25%–50% of the nucleus has to be removed, then widen the corneal main incision to 4 mm. Extract the nucleus fragments with the fragment forceps or a Vectis. Alternatively, you can inject viscoelastics (Viscoat®) behind the nuclear fragment so that it moves towards the main incision and then press with the viscoelastics cannula on to the lower lip of the main incision (viscoexpression). The fragments will now leave passively the anterior chamber. Do not use phacoemulsification. If you continue with phaco you risk dropping these nuclear fragments.

6. Injection of triamcinolone into the anterior chamber
7. Anterior vitrectomy and removal of cortex

The anterior vitrectomy can be performed from the limbus or from pars plana. We prefer and recommend working from pars plana.

First inject triamcinolone anterior and posterior to the iris to visualize the vitreous prolapse. Inject approximately 0.1 ml of diluted triamcinolone (30% triamcinolone and 70% BSS) into the anterior chamber. The triamcinolone crystals visualize the vitreous very well.

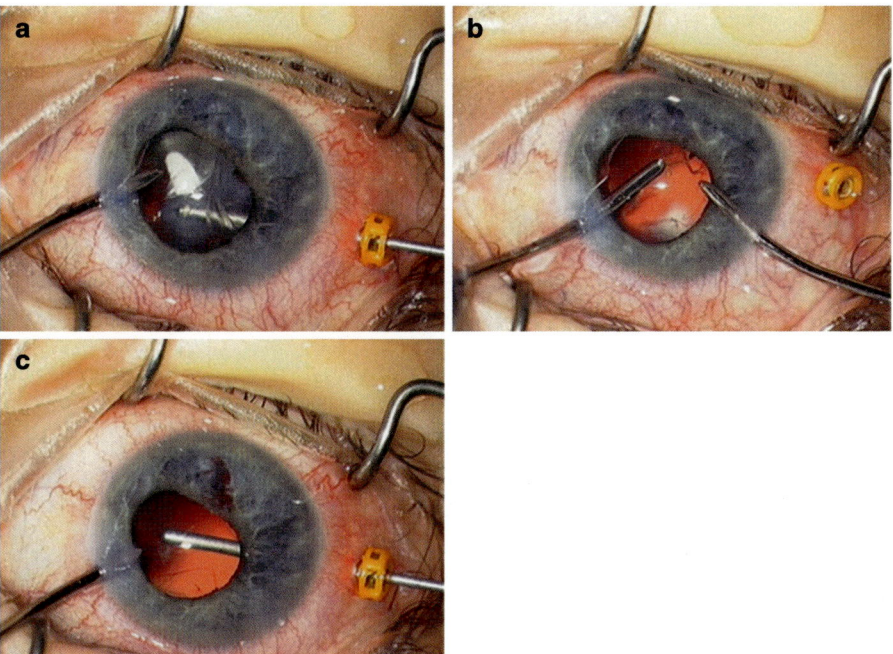

Fig. 13.8 (**a**): Place the infusion handpiece in the anterior chamber and begin with the anterior vitrectomy from pars plana. If epinucleus is present inside the lens capsule, then try to remove it first; it might drop otherwise into the vitreous cavity. (**b**) Then continue with removal of cortical cortex. You can use I/A for cortex removal but switch back to the vitreous cutter if you aspirate vitreous. (**c**) The tip of the vitreous cutter should always be visible when it moves behind the pupil. Cut the vitreous for approximately 5 min. The beginner tends to remove too little vitreous

Then start with anterior vitrectomy (Fig. 13.8). Regarding vitrectomy, the machine settings are important. We recommend the setting I/A-cut. Remove first the vitreous behind the capsular rupture (vitrectomy mode). Rotate the vitreous cutter port slowly in a circular fashion in order to remove as much vitreous body as possible. As a beginner, you tend to remove too little anterior vitreous; you need approximately 5 min for complete removal of the anterior vitreous. The visualisation of the vitreous with triamcinolone is a good help. Then carefully remove the remaining cortex with I/A handpieces. During this manoeuvre you have to switch between vitrectomy and aspiration back and forth because a vitreous prolapse may reoccur. This maneuver can also be performed with a vitreous cutter. When removing cortex use the vitrector only in aspiration mode. If you accidentally activate the vitrectomy mode during removal of the cortex, you will injure the anterior capsule.

8. Removal of Vitreous Strand

Check with a manipulator or an iris spatula, if a vitreous strand is present. An oval pupil is a sign for a vitreous strand. We recommend to visualize the vitreous with triamcinolone (Fig. 13.9). The vitreous strands are incarcerated into the cor-

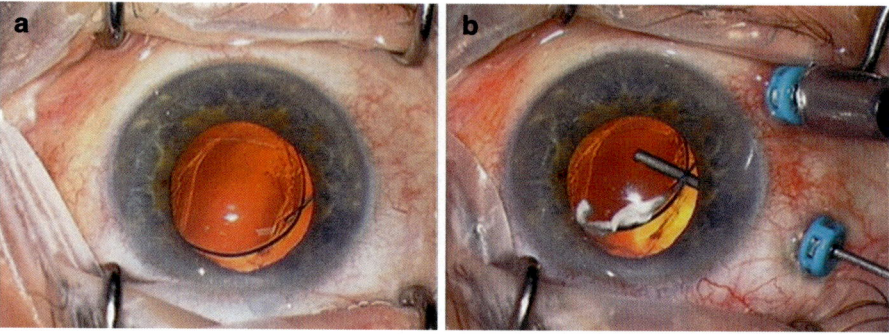

Fig. 13.9 (**a**) Is the vitreous completely removed? (**b**) Stain with triamcinolone and you will be surprised. There is vitreous!

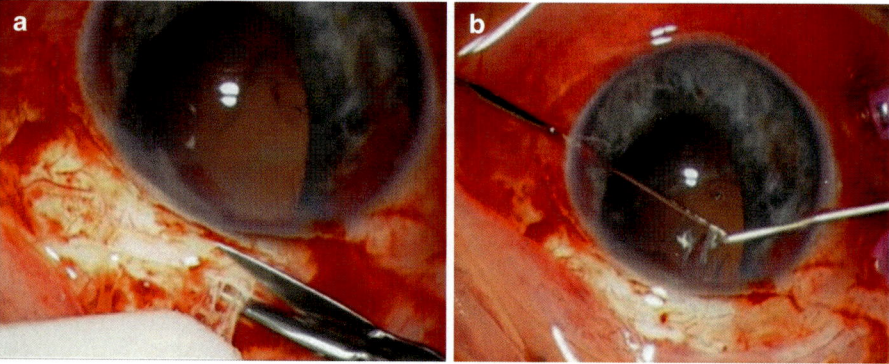

Fig. 13.10 (**a**) Note the vitreous prolapse through the main incision, stained with triamcinolone. It is removed with a cotton swab and scissors. (**b**) For removal of vitreous strands work bimanual. An iris spatula fixates the vitreous strand and the vitreous cutter removes it

neal wounds (paracentesis or main incision) and can be identified by a distorted pupil. If necessary, inject again triamcinolone. The removal of vitreous strands is *not* possible from pars plana. The vitreous cutter is inserted through a side incision. The second hand holds an iris spatula. Insert a spatula instrument through a paracentesis and rotate it in a circular fashion in the complete anterior chamber and check especially the incision sites. Catch a vitreous strand with the iris spatula, move it inside the pupil and then cut it with the vitreous cutter (Fig. 13.10). Perform the same manoeuvre from the second paracentesis.

  9. Insert iris hooks
10. Implantation of the IOL in the sulcus

Insert iris hooks to visualize the anterior capsule. If the anterior capsule is intact then proceed with a sulcus implantation. Insert first iris hooks to visualize the anterior capsule. Then inject viscoelastics (Viscoat®) into the anterior chamber and into the sulcus. Implant a 3-piece IOL and place both haptics first on the iris and then rotate them one by one into the sulcus. *Remark*: If you place the leading haptic onto the anterior lens capsule instead on the iris then the haptic often dislocates into posterior capsular rent and the IOL may drop.

11. Removal of Trocar

Remove the trocar cannula and close the sclerotomy with anatomic forceps. Alternatively, put the cutter inside the cannula, then remove the cannula and then pull the cutter in order to prevent vitreous wick. If the main incision was extended for the extraction of nuclear fragments, you should suture it with an Ethilon 10-0 cross stitch. Hydrate the side incisions and remove finally the trocar (Fig. 13.11).

Tips and Tricks
An alternative technique is IOL scaffolding (Fig. 13.12). This technique is applicable for any size of remaining lens fragments in case of posterior capsule break. It reduces the risk for loss of lens fragments into the vitreous cavity. Place the remain-

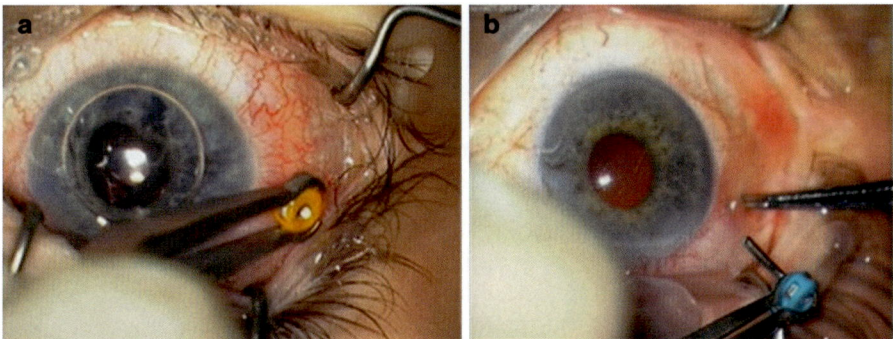

Fig. 13.11 (**a**) Inject an air bubble to stabilize the anterior chamber if necessary and remove finally the trocar with anatomic forceps or a trocar forceps. (**b**) Compress the wedges of the sclerotomy with the forceps for a few seconds. Remark: Two different trocars are used in (**a, b**)

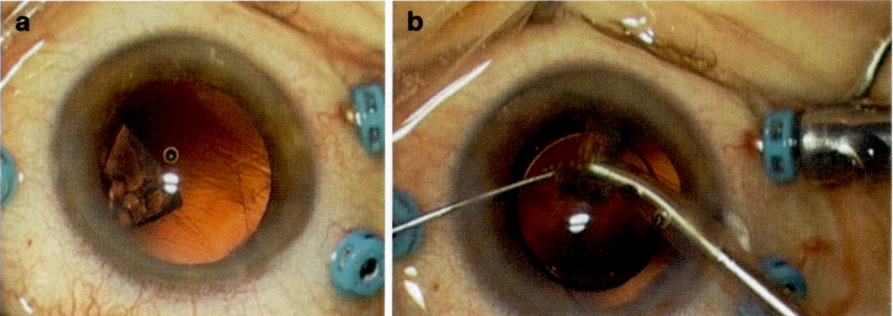

Fig. 13.12 (**a**) A nuclear fragment in an eye with PCR. (**b**) An IOL is placed inside the anterior chamber, the haptics rest on the iris. The nucleus fragment is located above the IOL and can be removed safely with the phaco handpiece

ing lens fragment in anterior chamber angle and then implant the IOL in the sulcus or over iris. The lens fragment is located on top of the IOL.

Another alternative technique is a sheet glide (no Figure). Use of sheet glide is advisable if using a 6 mm SICS main incision. The viscoexpression is easier.

Tips and Tricks

Postoperative distorted pupil with *incarcerated vitreous strand.* A vitreous strand should be removed because it causes a distorted pupil, a vitreous wick syndrome with an increased risk of infection and vitreous dragging with Irvine Gass syndrome or retinal tears. There are different methods:

1. This maneuver is performed at the slit lamp. Attach a 27G cannula to a 3 cc syringe. Insert the cannula opposite to the vitreous strand through the clear cornea and relieve the vitreous strand with a circular movement. The strand remains in the anterior chamber but causes no traction.
2. Use YAG vitreolysis after 2–3 weeks. The vitreous strand contracts and is more visible. It is safe to place a YAG contact lens on the cornea after 2–3 weeks.
3. Anterior vitrectomy. Remove the vitreous strand with the vitreous cutter. Insert the vitreous cutter through a paracentesis opposite to the vitreous strand, catch the vitreous strand with the tip of the cutter. Then move the cutter over the pupil and cut the vitreous strand.

The technique of surgical management of a PCR with trocar cannula is summarized in the following drawing (Fig. 13.13):

Summary The management of a posterior capsular rent depends on the timing of the rupture. If the rupture happens during phacoemulsification, then convert to manual extraction of nuclear fragments then anterior vitrectomy. An alternative method is the IOL scaffolding. If the rupture happens during I/A then you can convert directly to anterior vitrectomy. Train yourself to perform an anterior vitrectomy from pars plana with a trocar.

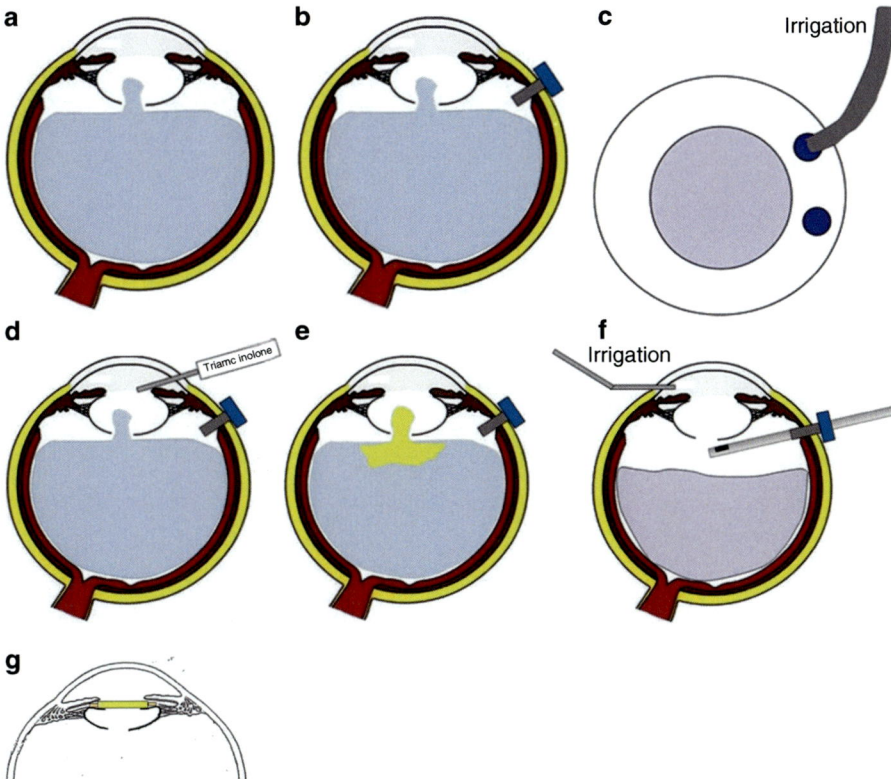

Fig. 13.13 Surgical management of a PCR with trocar cannulas. (**a**) PCR with vitreous prolapse. (**b**) Insertion of one trocar. (**c**) Insert infusion line or alternatively an anterior chamber maintainer. (**d**) Injection of triamcinolone (**e**) Triamcinolone stains the vitreous prolapse and the anterior vitreous (**f**) Removal of anterior vitreous from pars plana. For infusion use an irrigation handpiece, an anterior chamber maintainer or an infusion line with trocar cannula. (**g**) Sulcus implantation of IOL

Chapter 14
Surgical Technique of IOL Implantation in Eyes with Posterior Capsular Rent

The implantation of an IOL in an eye with posterior capsular rent (PCR) is difficult. The first step is assessment of the lens capsule and the second step is the surgery. The most important point of assessment is whether the anterior lens capsule is intact. If it is intact, then surgery is easy. The most important point of surgery is the insertion of iris hooks to fully visualize the anterior lens capsule and facilitate IOL implantation.

14.1 Sulcus Implantation with Intact Anterior Capsule

A sulcus implantation is required, if a posterior capsular rent (PCR) is present. What is the sulcus? The sulcus is the space between the iris and the anterior lens capsule (Fig. 14.1). A sulcus implantation requires an intact anterior lens capsule. If the anterior capsule is defect, then sulcus implantation is difficult. For details see following chapter.

A sulcus implantation requires a three-piece IOL. A one-piece IOL is not recommended because the thick haptics cause a depigmentation of the iris pigment (iris chaffing) resulting in a pigmentary glaucoma (Fig. 14.2).

I recommend warmly the insertion of iris hooks for examination and surgery. After insertion of iris hooks you can visualize and examine the anterior lens capsule (Fig. 14.1). Check if a rift or a zonular lysis is present. If not, you can proceed with surgery. Inject viscoelastics (Viscoat®) into the anterior chamber and into the sulcus. Then implant the IOL. Try to place the leading haptic on the iris. Then rotate the trailing haptic into the anterior chamber and place it also on the iris. Then rotate one haptic into the sulcus on top of the anterior capsule. Then rotate the second haptic

Electronic Supplementary Material The online version of this chapter (https://doi.org/10.1007/978-3-030-36093-1_14) contains supplementary material, which is available to authorized users.

U. Spandau, *Trocar Surgery for Cataract Surgeons*,
https://doi.org/10.1007/978-3-030-36093-1_14

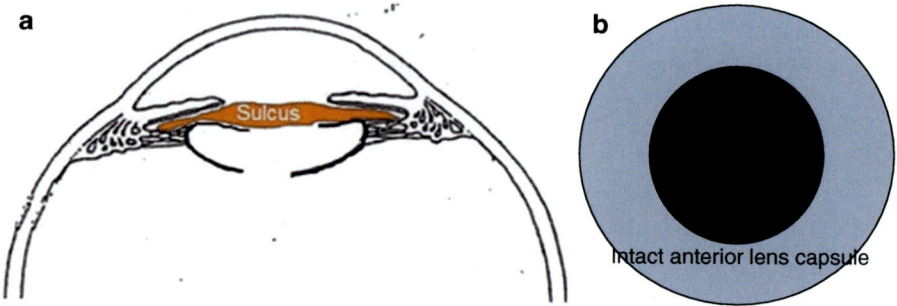

Fig. 14.1 (**a**) The sulcus is localized between iris and anterior lens capsule. (**b**) A sulcus implantation requires an intact anterior capsule. Insert iris hooks to visualize the anterior capsule

Fig. 14.2 Iris depigmentation secondary to implantation of a 1-piece IOL into the sulcus

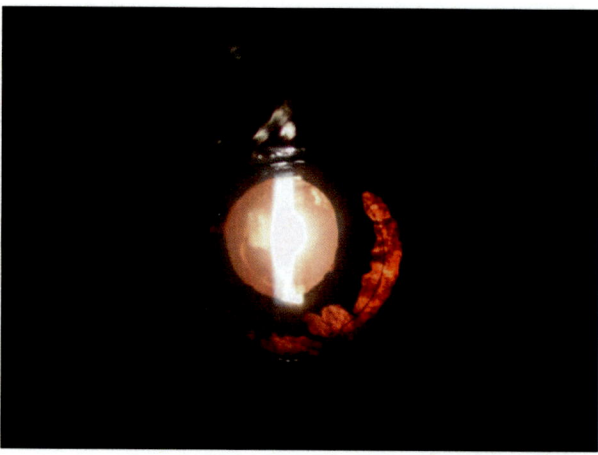

into the sulcus. If the rhexis is not too big you can perform an optic-in and haptic-out maneuver (optic capture by the capsulorhexis). The surgical technique is described in the next section. Finally remove first the iris hooks and then viscoelastics.

Surgery of IOL Capture Step-by-Step

In case of a posterior capsule tear, the best position for an IOL is "optic in, haptic out" (lens capture). The haptics are in the sulcus and the optic behind the rhexis of the anterior capsule (Fig. 14.3). The IOL is well centered, the iris-lens diaphragm is stabilized and the IOL is less myopic than in the sulcus. Another advantage relates to retinal surgery: a tamponade in the vitreous cavity cannot enter the anterior chamber.

Remark For lens capture the rhexis has to be well centered and slightly less in size than the IOL optic diameter.

Instrumentation

1. 2x manipulators (e.g. push-pull, Sinskey hook)

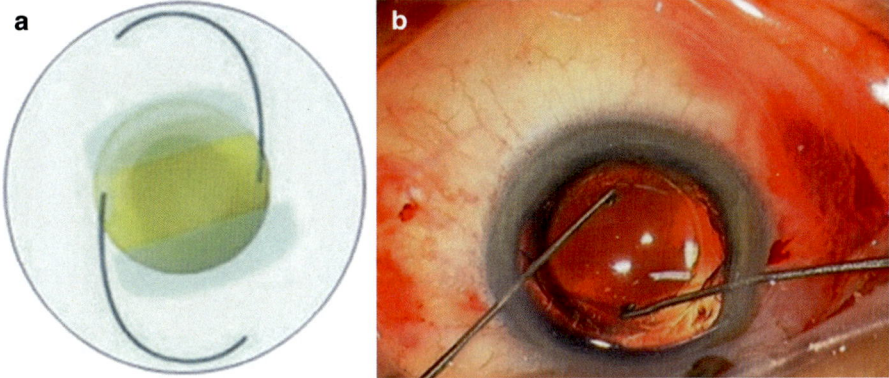

Fig. 14.3 (**a**) Drawing of a lens capture. The posterior capsule is defective. The IOL is placed in the sulcus and the optic is buttonholed behind the rhexis. The haptics remain in the sulcus. The round rhexis takes an almond shape. (**b**) Lens capture manoeuvre. Work bimanually with two Sinskey hooks or iris spatulas and press the optic at one side behind the rhexis while stabilizing the optic at the other side. Then the same manoeuvre at the other side

Procedure Two paracentesis at an angle of about 90 degrees to the haptics. If the haptics are located at 12 and 6 o'clock, then place the paracentesis at 3 and 9 o'clock. Take two Sinskey hooks (alternatively spatula), one Sinskey hook presses one side of the IOL behind the anterior capsule, while the other Sinskey hook stabilizes the IOL (Fig. 14.3). Then the same manoeuvre on the other side. Then examine with the push-pull instruments whether the rhexis margins are located before the IOL. When properly performed the rhexis takes an oval shape (Fig. 14.3).

14.2   Sulcus Implantation with Defect Anterior Capsule

The Videos 14.1 and 14.2 demonstrate the surgical management of a sulcus implantation.

Sulcus implantation becomes difficult when a rift is present. A haptic may dislocate through the rift resulting in a dislocation of the complete IOL.

We start with the same procedure. Insert 4 iris hooks and examine the anterior capsule. Where is the rift located? If the rift is located at 6 o'clock, then you must place the haptics in a diagonal way (Fig. 14.4). It may, however, happen that a haptic rotates during the postoperative course towards 6 o'clock and the IOL dislocates.

The IOL is safer, if the rift is located at 3 or 9 o'clock. In this case the IOL can be placed in the 12 and 6 o'clock position. A dislocation in the postoperative course is very unlikely (Fig. 14.5).

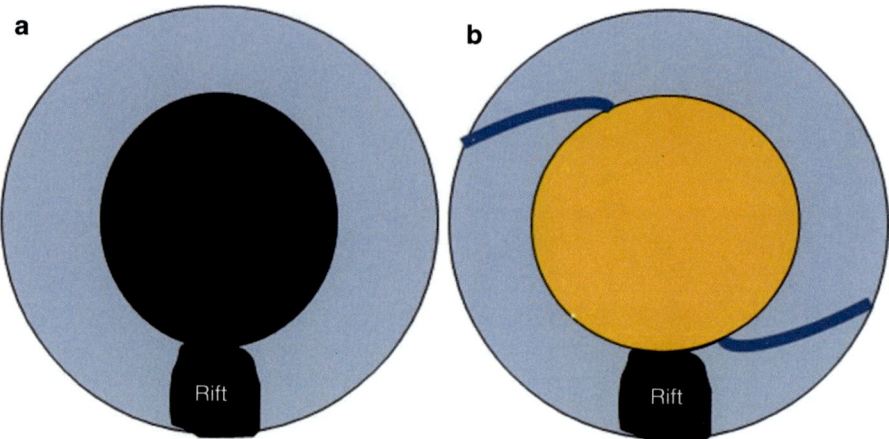

Fig. 14.4 (**a**) A rift at 6 o'clock. (**b**) Place the haptics in a diagonal position away from the 6 o'clock rift

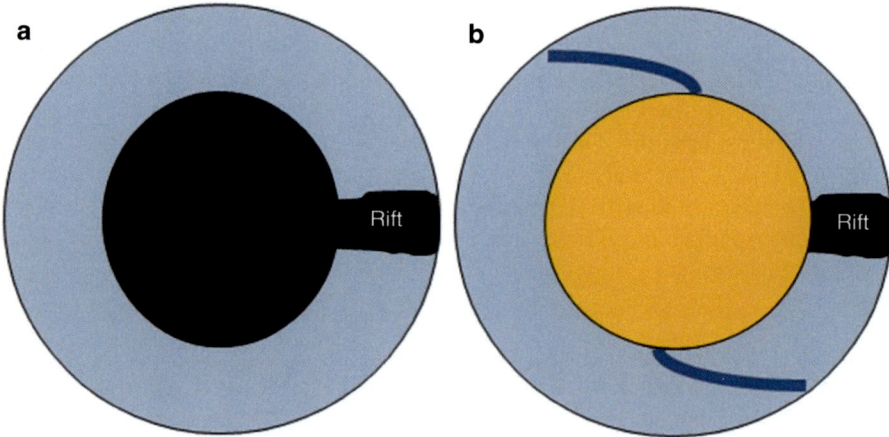

Fig. 14.5 (**a**) A rift at 3 or 9 o'clock. (**b**) Place the IOL with the haptics in the 6 and 12 o'clock position. Principle is to place the haptics away from the rift and at a maximum distance possible from the rift

14.3   In-the-Bag Implantation with Defect Posterior Capsule

In case of a PCR, it is possible to implant an IOL into the lens capsule. An IOL implantation inside the lens capsule is better than a sulcus position. Why? An IOL in sulcus position can rotate and is never stable. In contrast, an IOL in the lens capsule is stable and cannot rotate. If a vitreoretinal surgery is planned, then a gas tamponade may dislocate the IOL and in case of a silicone oil tamponade the silicone oil may prolapse into the anterior chamber if an IOL is placed in sulcus.

An in-the-bag implantation is, however, only possible if the PCR is located in the middle of the lens capsule (Fig. 14.6). If the PCR is located in the periphery of the lens capsule, then an in-the-bag implantation is not possible because the second haptic cannot be positioned safely (Fig. 14.7).

If you have much experience with the vitreous cutter, then you can perform a "PCR-plasty". Transform sharp edges to round edges with the vitreous cutter. Doing this you can transform an unstable PCR to a stable and round posterior capsular rhexis (Fig. 14.8). But a "PCR-plasty" is not required for in-the-bag implantation.

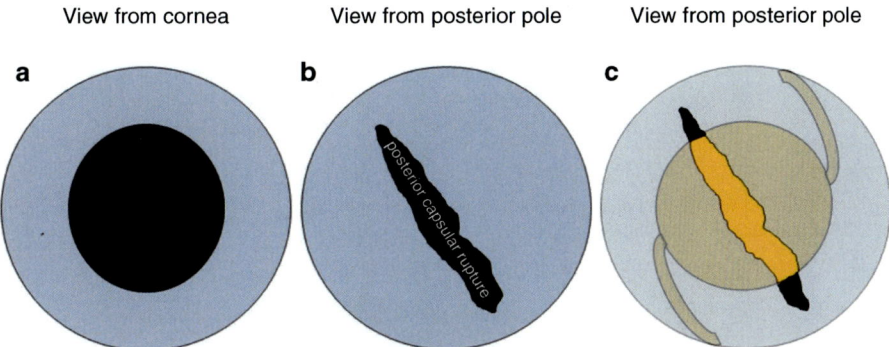

Fig. 14.6 (**a**) The anterior capsule is intact. (**b**) If the PCR is located in the middle of the posterior capsule then an in-the-bag implantation of the IOL is possible. (**c**) The haptics can be placed in the intact parts of the lens capsule

Fig. 14.7 If, however, the PCR is located in the periphery of the posterior capsule then an in-the-bag implantation of the IOL is difficult because one haptic is located in the PCR. A sulcus implantation has to be done instead

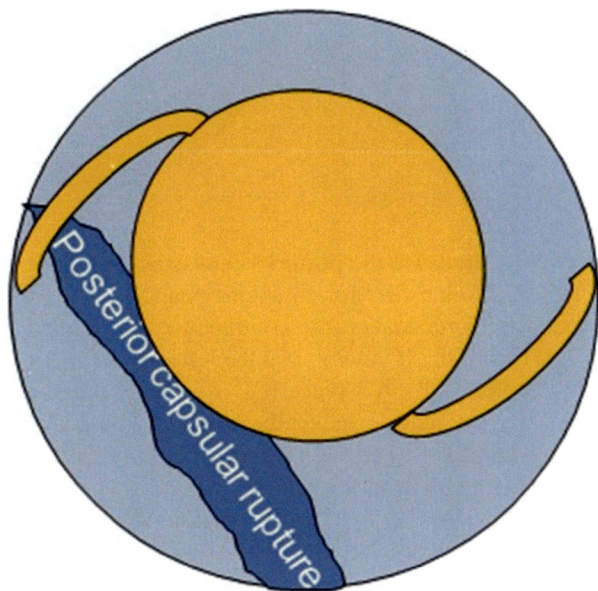

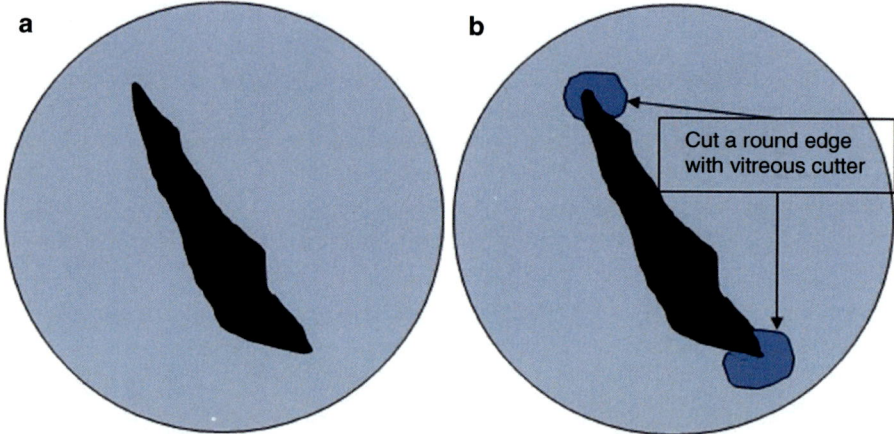

Fig. 14.8 The sharp edges of the PCR can tear out to the periphery of the lens capsule (**a**). Try to create a round edge with the vitreous cutter (**b**). The round edge transforms the unstable PCR to a stable circular posterior rhexis

Fig. 14.9 The zonules prevent that a rift in the anterior or posterior lens capsule continues over the lens equator to the other side

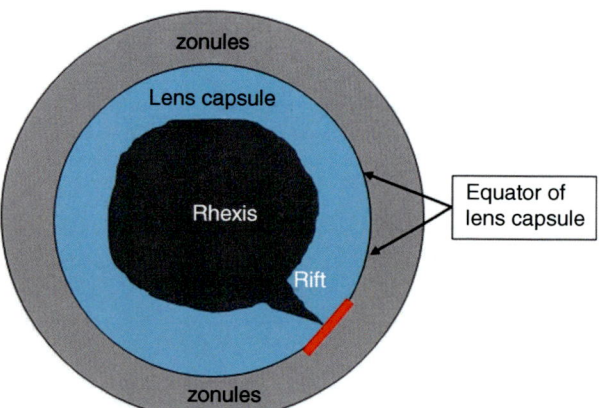

Why? Because the posterior lens capsule rupture (usually) stops at the zonules. This is also the case for an anterior capsular rift which stops at the zonules unless excessive force makes it to continue to the posterior lens capsule (Fig. 14.9).

Which IOL? If you implant the IOL inside the lens capsule, you can use a 1-piece or a 3-piece IOL. A 1-piece IOL is easier to implant inside the lens capsule. If you, however, are indecisive whether you will implant the IOL inside the lens capsule or inside the sulcus then use a 3-piece IOL. A 3-piece IOL can be implanted in the lens capsule as well as in the sulcus.

Chapter 15
Surgical Management of Zonular Lysis

The Videos 15.1 and 15.2 demonstrate the surgical management of a zonular lysis.

During cataract surgery a peripheral vitreous prolapse may occur secondary to a zonular lysis. There is no posterior capsular rent (PCR) present. The vitreous prolapses through the area of zonular defect into the anterior chamber (Fig. 15.1). This vitreous prolapse can only be removed from pars plana (Fig. 15.1b). Stain the vitreous prolapse from the anterior chamber with triamcinolone to assess the extent of vitreous prolapse.

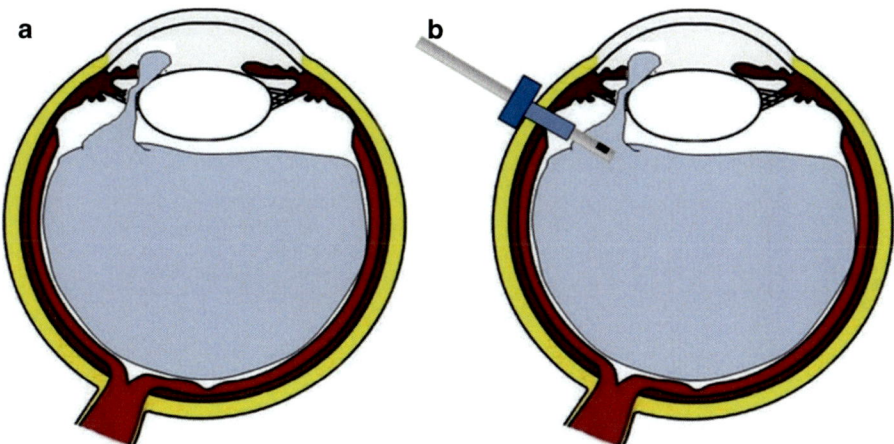

Fig. 15.1 (**a**) Vitreous prolapse secondary to zonular lysis. (**b**) The vitreous can only be removed from pars plana

Electronic Supplementary Material The online version of this chapter (https://doi.org/10.1007/978-3-030-36093-1_15) contains supplementary material, which is available to authorized users.

15.1   Cataract Surgery with Zonular Lysis

A cataract with zonular lysis is the most difficult cataract to operate (Fig. 15.2). Always check during the preoperative assessment, if a phacodonesis is present or not. If you are a beginner, you should rather send the patient to a hospital with retinal backup. The nucleus may drop and you should, therefore, be capable to convert to a SICS and to save a dropping nucleus from pars plana. See treatment algorithm (Fig. 15.3). If you note a zonular lysis after starting your

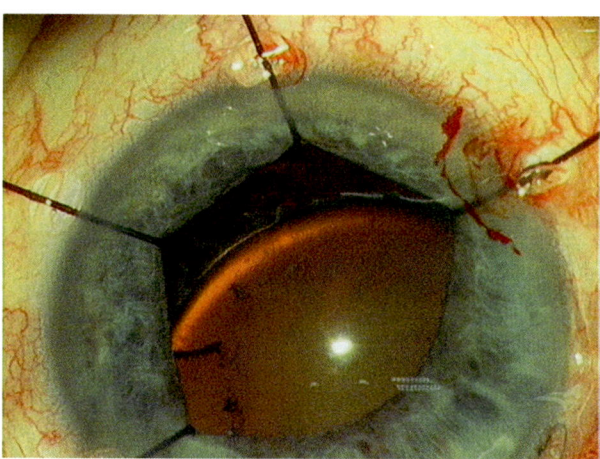

Fig. 15.2 A large zonular lysis secondary to pseudoexfoliation. After insertion of iris hooks the extent of the zonular lysis is visible

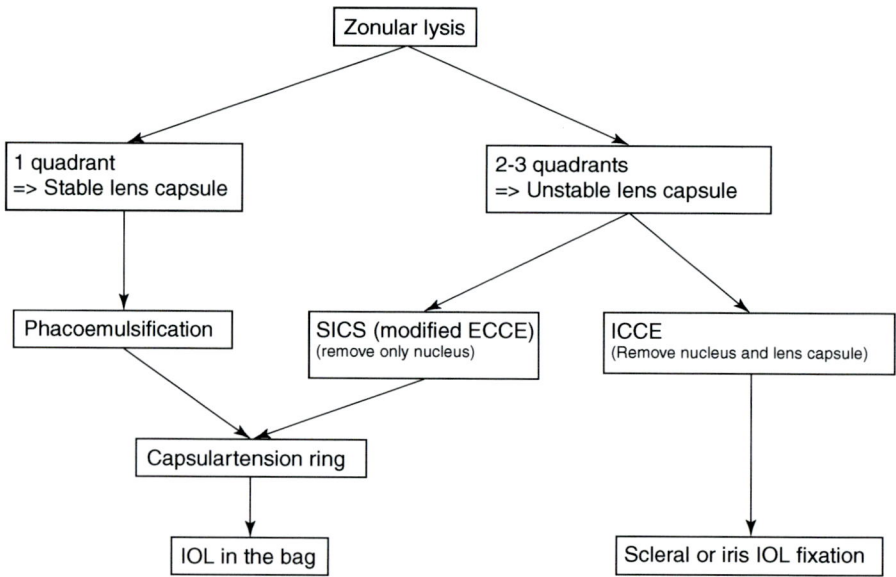

Fig. 15.3 Treatment algorithm for zonular lysis

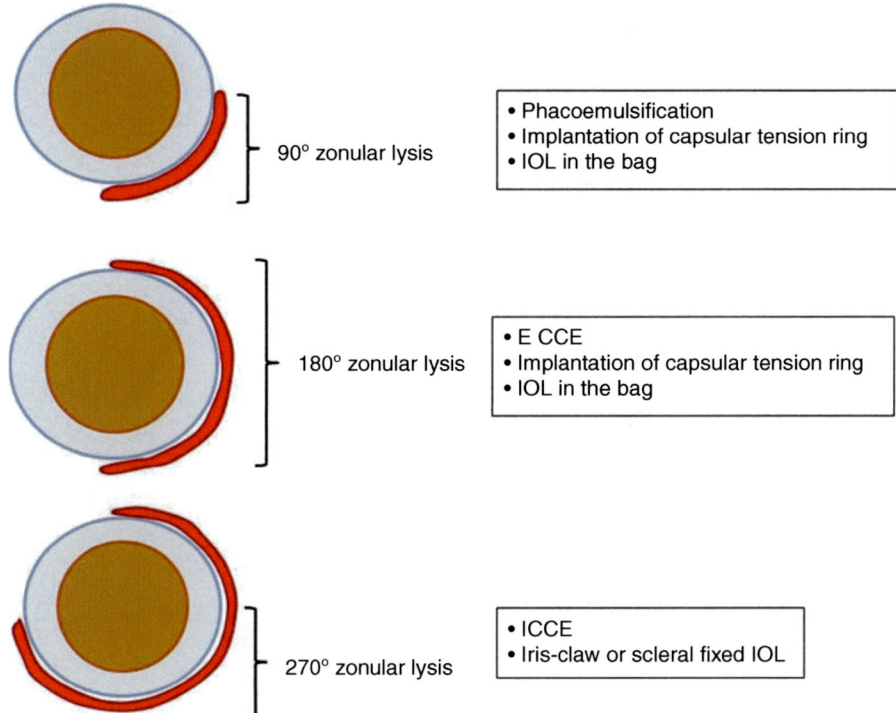

90° zonular lysis

- Phacoemulsification
- Implantation of capsular tension ring
- IOL in the bag

180° zonular lysis

- E CCE
- Implantation of capsular tension ring
- IOL in the bag

270° zonular lysis

- ICCE
- Iris-claw or scleral fixed IOL

Fig. 15.4 Treatment algorithm for zonular lysis. Depending on the size of the zonular lysis different surgical techniques are recommended

cataract case, then first assess the extent of the zonular lysis (Fig. 15.2). Insert iris hooks and inject triamcinolone to assess the size of the zonular lysis and the amount of vitreous prolapse.

A moderate zonular lysis of 1 quadrant is often discovered under I/A. Implant a capsular tension ring after I/A or insert the IOL with one haptic pressing against the loose quadrant.

If the zonular lysis is very advanced (2–3 quadrants), we prefer to perform a SICS (modified ECCE). A phacoemulsification on this situation is technically very difficult and risk full. See treatment algorithm (Fig. 15.4).

15.2 Zonular Lysis of One Quadrant

Instrumentation
Maybe: Iris retractors (Fig. 15.5)
  Capsular tension ring (Fig. 15.6)

Fig. 15.5 Iris hook (blue) with
a silicone stopper (transparent).
The iris hook grasps the
pupillary edge or the rhexis
edge and the silicone stopper
fixates the hook. Indication:
Small pupil or zonular lysis

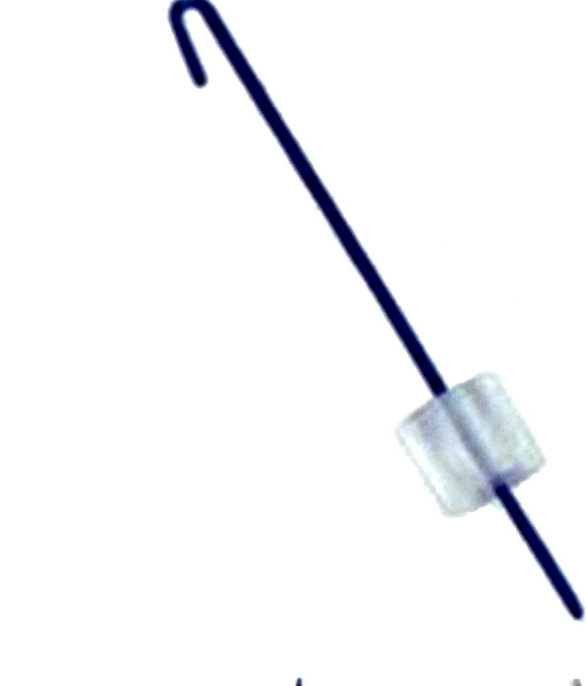

Fig. 15.6 A preloaded
capsular tension ring.
Indication: Zonular lysis
(Croma, Austria)

Individual Steps
1. Rhexis
2. Phacoemulsification
3. I/A
4. Implantation of capsular tension ring
5. Implantation of IOL in capsular bag

The Surgery Step-by-Step
1. Rhexis
2. Phacoemulsification
3. I/A

If you detect or suspect the zonular lysis under phacoemulsification, then continue
with as little stress on the zonules as possible. Don't press with the phaco tip on the
nucleus because pressure on the capsular bag increases the zonular lysis. Reduce
also the height of the bottle as much as possible.

4. Implantation of capsular tension ring
5. Implantation of IOL in capsular bag

Two possible *timings* for implantation of capsular tension ring: (1) As soon as you notice the zonular lysis. The advantage is a stable capsular bag. The disadvantage of an early implantation is that the cortex is difficult to remove because the capsular tension ring presses against the cortex. (2) After removal of the cortex. Advantage: Easy removal of cortex (Fig. 15.7).

We recommend to wait as long as possible with implantation of capsular tension ring.

Tips and Tricks
If you have already implanted CTR before cortex removal then try to remove the cortex by pulling cortex tangentially and not pulling centrally.

Procedure Inflate the capsular bag with viscoelastics (Viscoat®). Inject the capsular tension ring with an injector (Figs. 15.8 and 15.9). Be cautious that you place the

Fig. 15.7 A traumatic cataract with 1 quadrant zonular lysis

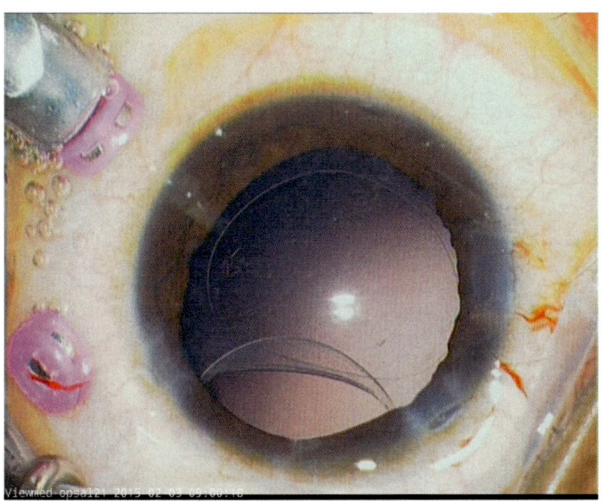

Fig. 15.8 A preloaded capsular tension ring in action

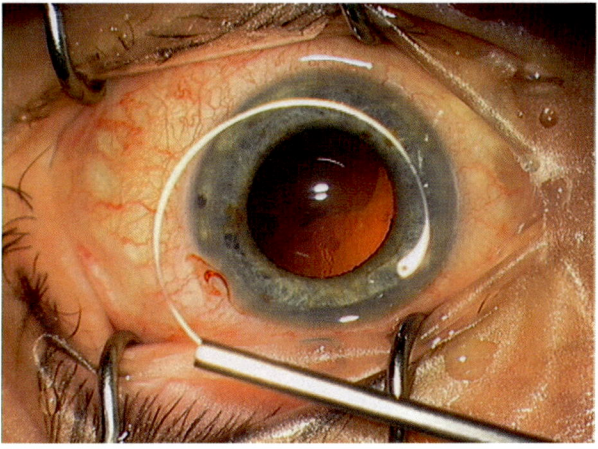

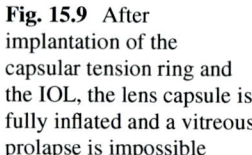
Fig. 15.9 After implantation of the capsular tension ring and the IOL, the lens capsule is fully inflated and a vitreous prolapse is impossible

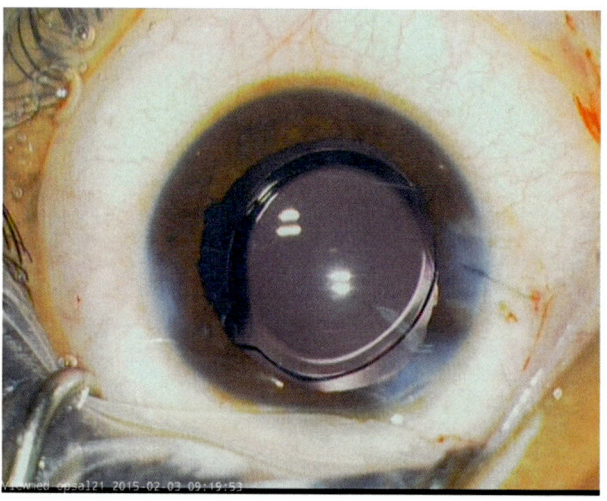

tip in the capsular bag and not in the sulcus. If you have placed the CTR in the bag, the folds in posterior capsule starts flattening as the bag gets stretched.

Alternatively, you can implant the IOL so that one haptic presses against the zonular lysis and thereby fully inflating the lens capsule. It is important that the lens capsule is completely inflated in order to prevent vitreous prolapse.

15.3   Zonular Lysis of Two Quadrants

If you try to remove the nucleus with the phacoemulsification handpiece then the risk is high that the complete lens with capsule drops into the vitreous cavity. Why? Because phacoemulsification causes additional stress on the zonules and may result in a dropped nucleus. In addition, if you increase the zonular lysis during phaco-emulsification then an in-the-bag implantation will not be possible. Technically much easier and less risk full is a SICS (modified ECCE). The nucleus is luxated from the lens capsule and placed onto the iris and then extracted through a scleral incision. This technique causes minimal stress on the zonules and an IOL-in-the-bag implantation is possible in most cases.

Instruments
1. Caliper
2. 15° knife
3. 2.4 mm tunnel knife
4. Crescent bevel-up knife
5. Lens extraction hook (Geuder No: 32034, Germany); *alternative*: serrated lens loop

Material
1. Iris retractors
2. Capsular tension ring
3. 3-piece IOL or PMMA IOL

Individual Steps
1. Large capsular rhexis
2. Frown incision
3. Luxation of the nucleus into the anterior chamber
4. Extraction of the nucleus
5. I/A
6. Implantation of a capsular tension ring
7. Implantation of a 3-piece IOL
8. Closure of the frown incision and conjunctiva

The Surgery Step-by-Step
1. Large capsular rhexis
2. Frown incision

In case of a small pupil insert iris hooks in order to obtain a large rhexis. Perform a large circular rhexis. If the lens capsule is very unstable you can insert now the iris hooks into the rhexis margin (Fig. 15.10). Continue with the frown incision. Perform a limbal peritomy from 11 to 1 o'clock with Westcott scissors and cauterize the bleeding vessels. Then mark an 8 mm wide incision with a caliper. The incision should be 1–1.5 mm behind the limbus. Continue with a frown incision with a 15° knife (50% scleral thickness). Then dissect a scleral tunnel with the crescent angled bevel up knife (Fig. 15.11).

3. Luxation of the nucleus into the anterior chamber
4. Extraction of the nucleus

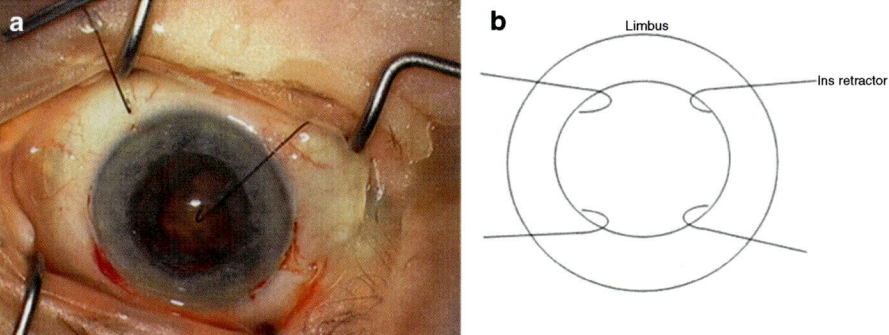

Fig. 15.10 (**a**) The iris hooks are placed in the rhexis edge. (**b**) Drawing of the implantation of iris hooks in the rhexis edge in case of a zonular lysis

Fig. 15.11 Dissect a
scleral flap for the frown
incision. The incision is
8 mm wide

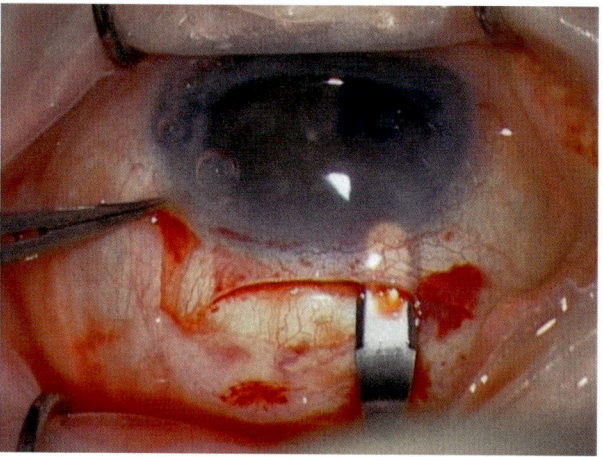

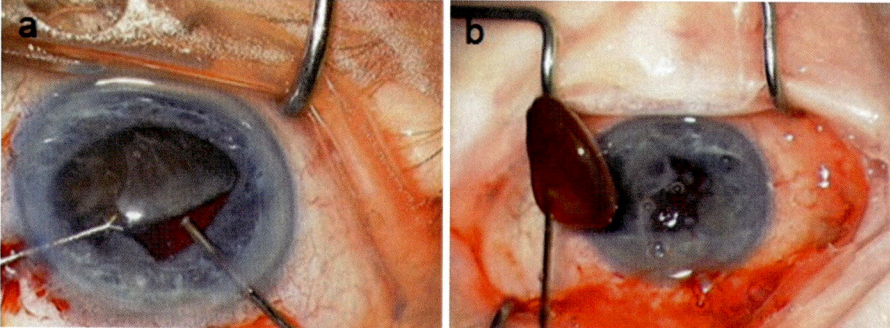

Fig. 15.12 (**a**) Lift the nucleus up with a nucleus manipulator (y-hook) and inject at once visco-elastic between nucleus and posterior lens capsule. (**b**) Extract the nucleus with a fish hook or a lens loop

Continue by luxating the nucleus bimanually with 2 manipulators (e.g. push-pull or Rosen chopper and viscoelastics cannula) into the anterior chamber (Fig. 15.12). Then use the lens extraction hook or a lens loop. Proceed by placing the tip of the vectis (lens hook, lens loop) behind the center of the nucleus and then extract the nucleus with the lens hook (Fig. 15.12). If the nucleus gets stuck in the main incision, you have to extend it. After removal of the nucleus you can express residual cortical material with viscoexpression.

5. I/A
6. Implantation of a capsular tension ring
7. Implantation of an iris-fixated IOL

Then continue with I/A and remove the cortex. This manoeuvre is of course difficult due to zonular lysis. Implant therefore at once or after I/A a capsular tension ring (Fig. 15.13). I recommend getting acquainted with the capsular tension ring

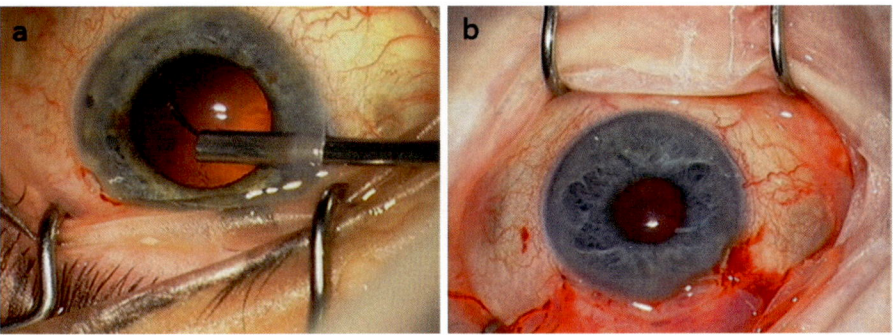

Fig. 15.13 (**a**) Inject a capsular tension ring to inflate the lens capsule and to prevent vitreous prolapsed. (**b**) Implant a 3-piece IOL or a PMMA IOL

before using it the first time. Then implant an IOL with or without injector into the lens capsule (Fig. 15.13).

Tips and Tricks
In case of *zonular lysis*, it is important to implant the IOL into the lens capsule and not into the sulcus because the IOL will luxate into the vitreous cavity if positioned in the sulcus.

8. Closure of frown incision and conjunctiva

Suture the frown incision with a Vicryl 8–0 cross stitch and the conjunctiva with one Vicryl 8–0 interrupted stitch. Inject cefuroxime (Zinacef®) intracameral as endophthalmitis prophylaxis.

Summary A large zonular lysis with hard nucleus is the most challenging case in cataract surgery. If you do not have retinal backup then avoid a phacoemulsification. A phacoemulsification is very risk full. Extract the nucleus with SICS (modified ECCE), implant a capsular tension ring and implant the IOL inside the lens capsule.

15.4 Zonular Lysis of Three Quadrants

If three quadrants are affected than it is advisable to remove the nucleus and the lens capsule with an ICCE procedure. The surgery is identical to the nucleus removal surgery in the previous chapter (SICS procedure). The only difference is that the frown incision is larger. A 9–10 mm frown incision is required. For the extraction of the nucleus we recommend a serrated lens loop and not a fish hook because the nucleus is very unstable.

The Surgery Step-by-Step
1. 9–10 mm frown incision

For an ICCE a large frown incision is required.

2. Insertion of 1–2 trocar cannulas
3. Extraction of the nucleus

Inject viscoelastics into the anterior chamber. Insert the vitreous cutter through the trocar cannula and elevate the nucleus at 12 o'clock. Then insert the serrated lens loop and push it behind the nucleus. Then extract the nucleus. It is advisable to remove the nucleus together with the lens capsule (ICCE) in order to avoid loss of cortical fragments.

4. Anterior vitrectomy

The large frown incision creates an unstable globe. It is advisable to close the frown incision with a X-suture before continuing with anterior vitrectomy. Check that the globe has normal tension and look for vitreous prolapse at the main incision. Continue with an anterior vitrectomy from pars plana. The anterior vitreous can be visualized more easily with triamcinolone staining.

5. IOL implantation

In case of a traumatic nucleus removal we recommend a delayed IOL implantation. Otherwise, continue with an iris or sclera fixated IOL implantation.

6. Closure of frown incision with two X-sutures

Close the frown incision with two Vicryl 8–0 X-sutures.

Tips and Tricks
Removal of lens capsule: In case of completely unstable lens capsule remove the lens capsule with forceps, for example a 20G or 23G serrated jaws forceps (Fig. 15.14). Now you have to implant a scleral or iris fixated IOL.

Fig. 15.14 If the lens capsule is too unstable then extract it with serrated jaws forceps (Alcon or Dorc)

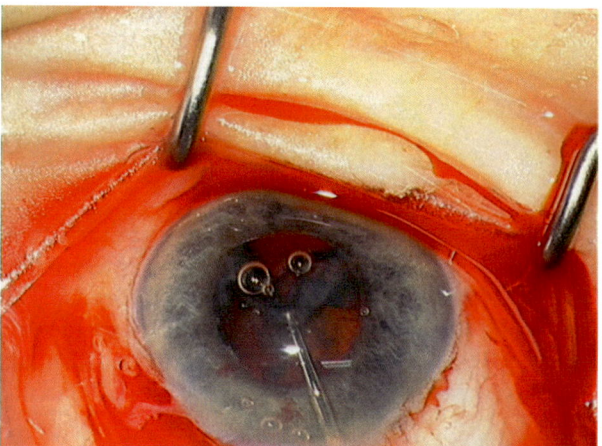

Chapter 16
Surgical Management of Anterior Dislocated IOL with Retropupillar Artisan Implantation

The Videos 14.2, 16.1, 16.2, 16.3, 16.4, and 16.5 demonstrate the surgical management of a dislocated IOL.

An IOL may dislocate on its own or together with the lens capsule (in-the-bag IOL) (Fig. 16.1a). Zonular lysis secondary to pseudoexfoliation is very common in Scandinavia. Many years after cataract surgery, an IOL may dislocate due to zonular lysis. The IOL's dislocate together with the lens capsule, a so called in-the-bag dislocation. In our hospital we operate approximately one patient per week due to dislocated IOL (Fig. 16.1b).

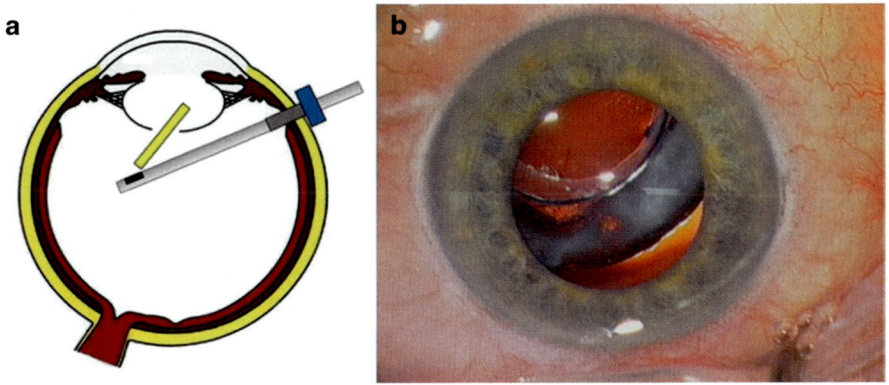

Fig. 16.1 (**a**) A dislocated IOL secondary to a posterior capsular rent. (**b**) A subluxated in-the-bag IOL secondary to zonular lysis. The IOL can be easily elevated from pars plana

Electronic Supplementary Material The online version of this chapter (https://doi.org/10.1007/978-3-030-36093-1_16) contains supplementary material, which is available to authorized users.

© Springer Nature Switzerland AG 2020
U. Spandau, *Trocar Surgery for Cataract Surgeons*,
https://doi.org/10.1007/978-3-030-36093-1_16

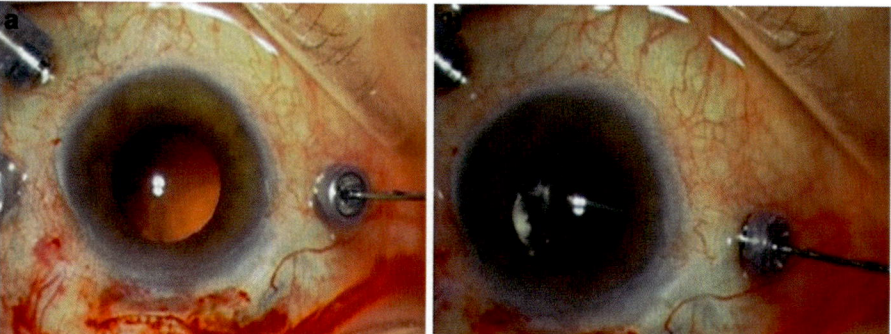

Fig. 16.2 (**a**) A dislocated IOL secondary to zonular lysis. The IOL cannot be elevated from the limbus into the anterior chamber. (**b**) After insertion of a trocar the IOL can be easily elevated with the viscoelastic cannula or vitreous cutter into the anterior chamber

In most cases a subluxated IOL cannot be reached from the limbus, but from pars plana it is easy to reach. Why? Because you can access the backside of the IOL from pars plana and then lift the IOL into the anterior chamber (Fig. 16.2).

Remark Subluxation: When the lens or IOL gets displaced but remains in the pupillary area. *Dislocation* or *luxation*: When the lens or IOL gets displaced and is out of the pupillary area.

In case of an in-the-bag IOL dislocation there are three possible IOL implantations. (1) Iris claw IOL, (2) anterior chamber IOL and (3) scleral fixated IOL. Anterior chamber IOL's are controversial because they cause endothelial cell loss and injure the iris root. In contrast, scleral fixated IOL's and here especially the Yamane technique are nowadays very popular. In this chapter I will demonstrate the third option, the implantation of an iris-claw IOL (Artisan) IOL.

The benefits of an iris claw IOL (Artisan) implantation are a short surgical time, a sutureless implantation, an excellent centration without risk of tilting and a short learning curve (approx. five surgeries). The surgical time is approximately 10 min. A redislocation happens seldom, maybe one patient per year. The disadvantage is that the IOL is fixated into the iris tissue and a too traumatic implantation may lead to an inflammation. This postoperative inflammation with cellular proliferation of the IOL is induced by macrophages. This occurs, however, only in the learning curve. If you combine the Artisan implantation with a complete PPV then a pseudophacodonesis may occur. If the Artisan implantation, however, is only combined with an anterior vitrectomy then the risk for a pseudophacodonesis is low.

In addition, sufficient iris tissue is required for implantation, e.g. an implantation in case of aniridia is not possible.

We will demonstrate the implantation of an iris claw IOL (Verisyse®, Abbott and Artisan®, Opthec) (Fig. 16.3). The iris claw IOL can be implanted before the pupil or behind the pupil. If you implant the IOL retropupillary then it has to be done "upside down" (= on the back) because the haptics are bent upwards.

Fig. 16.3 An iris-claw
IOL (Artisan®, Ophtec and
Verisyse®, AMO)

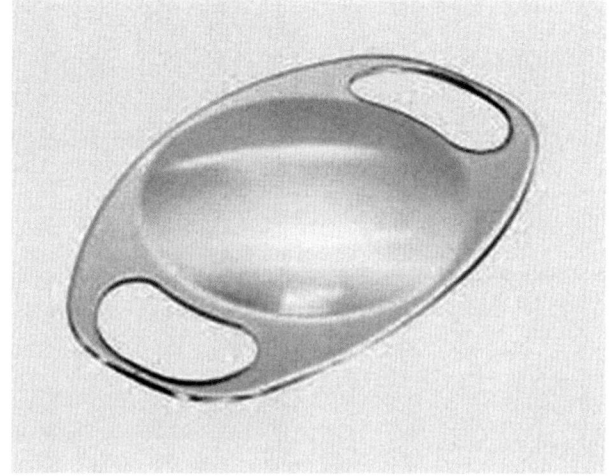

We will demonstrate the retropupillary method, which is easy to learn. We recommend starting with an aphakic eye which underwent an anterior vitrectomy. The pupil should be constricted before surgery. We recommend retrobulbar anesthesia.

There are different A-constants for antepupillar and retropupillar IOL implantations the A-constant for retropupillar implantation is 116.9.

The most difficult part of the surgery is the dissection of a scleral tunnel, which is the same as for the SICS technique (modified ECCE). We prefer a scleral tunnel to a corneal tunnel in order to reduce astigmatism; this tunnel is 6 mm wide. Why? Because the iris-claw IOL is 6 mm wide and because the extracted IOL is also 6 mm wide. What may happen if the tunnel is 8 mm wide? The wider the tunnel, the more you risk a choroidal detachment. In the beginning, we recommend starting with a 6 mm limbal tunnel. If you feel safe with the technique you can continue with a scleral tunnel.

How many trocars? We use usually only two trocars without a viewing system. We perform only an anterior vitrectomy and no core vitrectomy. A core vitrectomy increases te risk for pseudophacodonesis.

16.1   Special Instruments for Iris Claw IOL Implantation

Instruments for Iris Fixated IOL
The required instruments for the implantation of an iris-fixated IOL can be acquired from the company (Verisyse®, Abbott and Artisan®, Opthec).

IOL Implantation Forceps (Fig. 16.4)
Indication: Holds the Artisan (Verisyse IOL) during implantation. A very important instrument.

Fig. 16.4 Two instruments are required for the implantation of an Artisan IOL. (**a**) An IOL implantation forceps (AMO), (**b**) an enclavation spatula from Sekundo (Geuder) for implantation of an iris -claw IOL. Alternative: Iris spatula or anterior chamber cannula

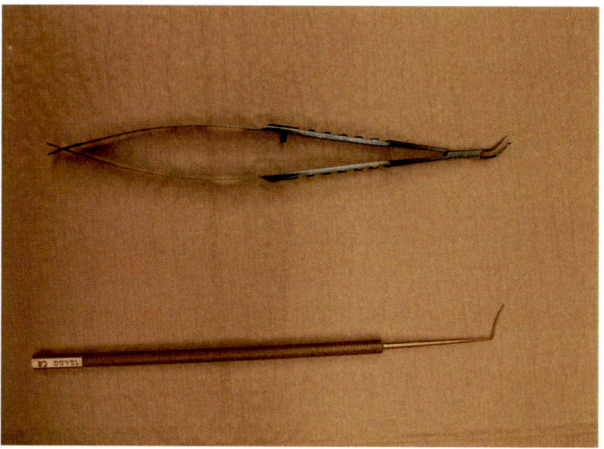

Fig. 16.5 Useful is also a Castroviejo's caliper. Indication: Frown incision (Geuder)

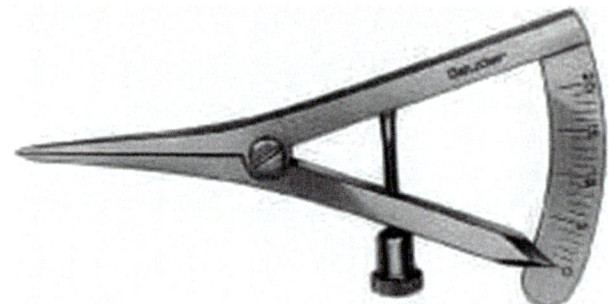

Enclavation Spatula (Fig. 16.4)

Indication: Retropupillar fixation of IOL-claws in iris tissue. This spatula is thin so that only a little iris tissue is enclavated. Sekundo enclavation spatula, Geuder-32,724.

Caliper (Fig. 16.5)

Indication: Marking of main incision and sclerotomy. The main incision for the implantation of an iris-fixated PMMA IOL is 6 mm wide. Caliper by Castroviejo, Geuder 19,135.

Serrated Jaw Forceps (Fig. 16.6)

Indication: Extraction of subluxated IOL with lens capsule. 20G or 23G. DORC. 1286.C06.

16.2   Iris Claw IOL Implantation Surgery

Instruments

1. Crescent bevel-up knife
2. 15° knife

Fig. 16.6 A 23G intravitreal serrated jaws forceps (DORC). Indication: Extraction of the subluxated IOL from the anterior chamber

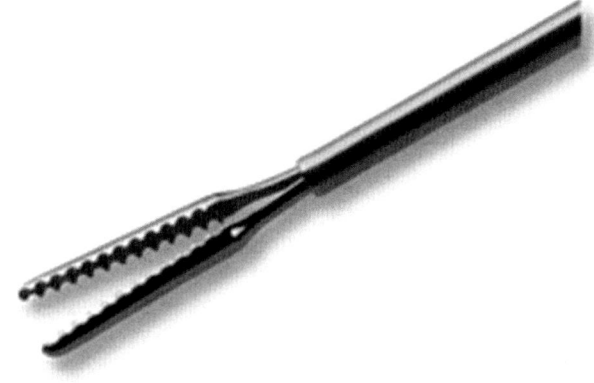

3. 2.4 mm tunnel knife
4. Caliper
5. IOL implantation forceps (AMO)
6. Enclavation spatula
7. 20G or 23G Serrated jaw forceps

Material
- Acetylcholine (Miochol)
- Iris claw IOL (Artisan®, Verisyse®)
- Maybe: Triamcinolone

Individual Steps
1. Two 23G trocars
2. Paracentesis at 3 and 9 o'clock
3. Limbal main incision/Scleral frown incision
4. Extraction of an anterior dislocated IOL
5. Anterior vitrectomy
6. Injection of Miochol
7. Implantation of iris fixated IOL (upside down)
8. Enclavation of iris fixated IOL
9. Closure of the frown incision and conjunctiva

The Surgery Step-by-Step: Figs. 16.7, 16.8, 16.9, 16.10, 16.11, 16.12, 16.13, and 16.14
1. Two 23G trocars.
2. Paracentesis at 3 and 9 o'clock.

Insert two trocars at the temporal side. Continue with a short paracentesis at 3 o'clock and 9 o'clock. The paracentesis is short so that you can reach the peripheral iris with the enclavation spatula.

Note The location of the IOL is determined by the position of the frown incision. If the claws are located at 3 o'clock and 9 o'clock, then the frown incision must be located at 12 o'clock. In case of an iris defect at 3 o'clock or a filtration bleb at 12 o'clock you must choose the position of the IOL and frown incision accordingly.

3. Limbal main incision/scleral frown incision.

Continue with the frown incision. Perform a limbal peritomy from 11 to 1 o'clock with Westcott scissors and cauterize the bleeding vessels (Fig. 16.7). Then mark a 6-mm wide incision (not wider!) with a caliper (Fig. 16.8). The arc of the incision should be approximately 1–2 mm behind the limbus. Dissect a 50% scleral thickness deep frown incision with a 15° knife (Fig. 16.9a). Then dissect a scleral tunnel with the crescent angled bevel up knife (Fig. 16.9b) and open finally the anterior chamber with a 2.4 mm blade (Fig. 16.10). Note: Enter the anterior chamber with the 2.4 mm blade in the clear cornea in order to avoid an intracameral bleeding and also to create a valve at the inner lip of the tunnel.

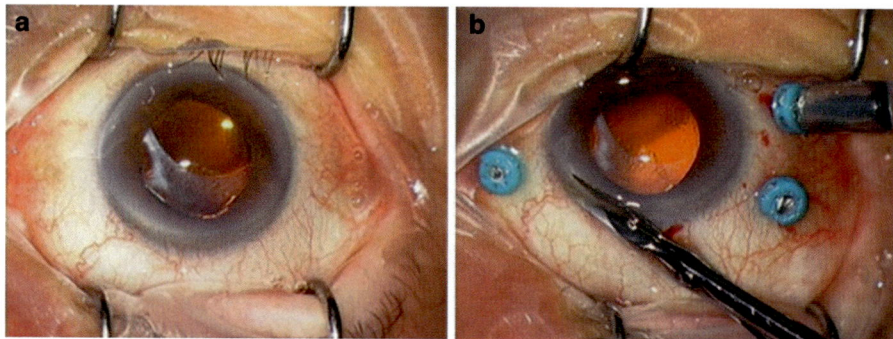

Fig. 16.7 (**a**) An anterior dislocated bag-IOL complex secondary to zonular lysis. (**b**) Open the conjunctiva along the limbus from 11 o'clock to 1 o'clock with the Vannas scissors (limbal peritomy)

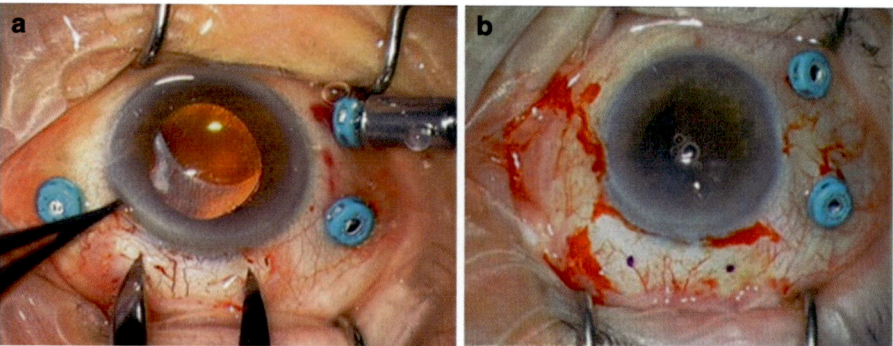

Fig. 16.8 (**a**) Mark a 6 mm broad scleral incision with the caliper. The incision is approximately 1.5 mm behind the limbus. (**b**) Mark the frown incision with a marker pen

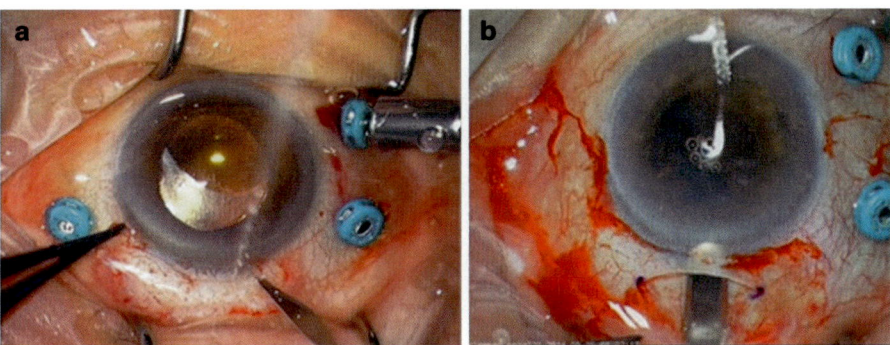

Fig. 16.9 (**a**) A 50% scleral thickness incision with the 15 deg. knife is performed. (**b**) Dissect a scleral tunnel with the bevel up crescent knife. If the knife is visible through the sclera, then you have the correct depth

Fig. 16.10 Then open the anterior chamber in the clear cornea with a 2.4 mm blade

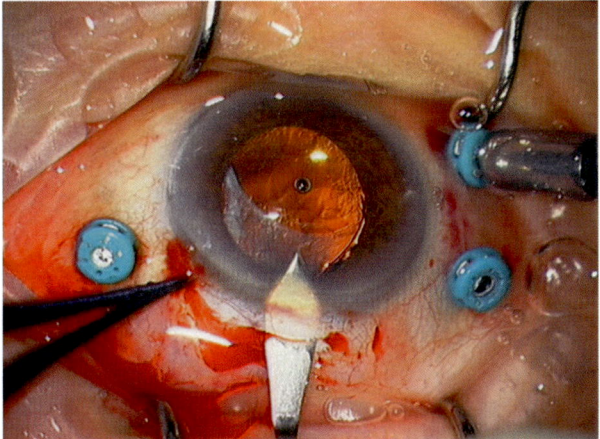

4. Extraction of an anterior dislocated IOL.

The extraction is easier, if the eye is not vitrectomized and the IOL is located behind the iris, Close the infusion line during extraction. Inject viscoelastics (Viscoat®) into the anterior chamber and then behind the IOL and elevate then the IOL a little bit up at 12 o'clock so that the optic edge or a haptic is visible (Fig. 16.11a). Grasp the IOL ideally at the haptic with the serrated jaw forceps and extract the IOL with the lens capsule (Fig. 16.11b). Often some fibrotic parts of the lens capsule remain in the anterior chamber. Remove them with viscoexpression, e.g. inject viscoelastics behind them into the anterior chamber and then press on the posterior scleral lip of the scleral tunnel; the fragment will leave the anterior chamber passively.

Reopen the infusion line and continue with an anterior vitrectomy from pars plana.

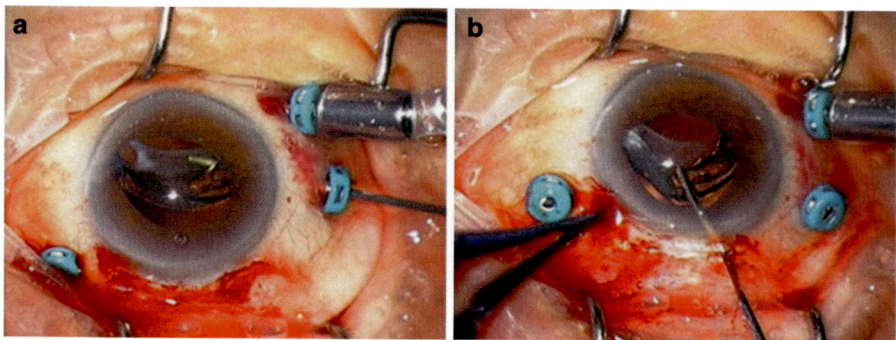

Fig. 16.11 (**a**) Prolapse the IOL at 12 o'clock up to the pupillary plane in order to access it with the forceps. (**b**) Then remove the IOL with the serrated jaws forceps

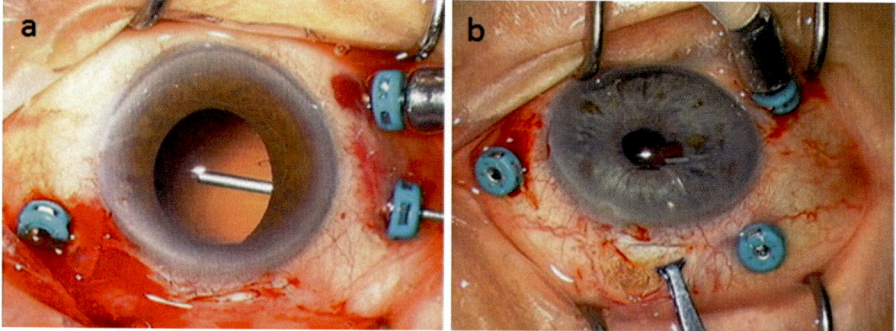

Fig. 16.12 (**a**) Perform an anterior vitrectomy. (**b**) Turn the iris-claw IOL upside down for implantation and implant it with the IOL implantation forceps (AMO)

5. Anterior vitrectomy.
6. Injection of Miochol.
7. Implantation of iris fixated IOL (upside down).

Continue with an anterior vitrectomy (Fig. 16.12). Move the tip of the vitreous cutter along the pupillary edge. The opening of the vitreous cutter points towards the optic disc. The next step is pupil constriction. Before implantation of an iris claw IOL, the pupil must be constricted. Inject first acetylchloline (Miochol®) and then viscoelastics (Viscoat®) to maintain anterior chamber. Using an IOL forceps (AMO) place the IOL *upside down* onto the iris. (Fig. 16.11). Then rotate the IOL so that the claws are located in the 3 and 9 o'clock position. Check the paracentesis with the Sekundo spatula. The view must be free in the area of the claws, remove blood if present. *Remark*: For retropupillar implantation the Artisan IOL is implanted upside down. Otherwise a basal iridectomy is required.

8. Enclavation of iris fixated IOL.

Instrumentation
- Dominant hand: IOL implantation forceps (Abbott).
- Non-dominant hand: Enclavation spatula.

Close the infusion line during IOL implantation. Centrate the IOL with a manipulator (e.g. push-pull) inside the anterior chamber. Grasp the IOL at the superior edge with the IOL implantation forceps (Abbott) (Fig. 16.13a). Flip the IOL to the right (Fig. 16.13b) so that half of the IOL is behind the iris and then to flip it to the left so that the IOL is completely behind the iris. Hold the IOL now in the middle of the pupil. Do not move it to the left or right.

Take then the enclavation spatula in your left hand. Lift the IOL a little bit up, so that the iris claws make an elevated impression behind the iris tissue. Then insert the spatula in the 3 o'clock paracentesis and clamp the iris tissue between the iris-claws (Fig. 16.13c). Then the hands for the implantation forceps have to be switched. This maneuver should be practiced preoperatively. Then take the enclavation spatula in your right hand and perform the same maneuver at 9 o'clock (Fig. 16.13d). Remove finally the implantation forceps and open the infusion line to achieve normotension. A retropupillary implantation requires no iridectomy.

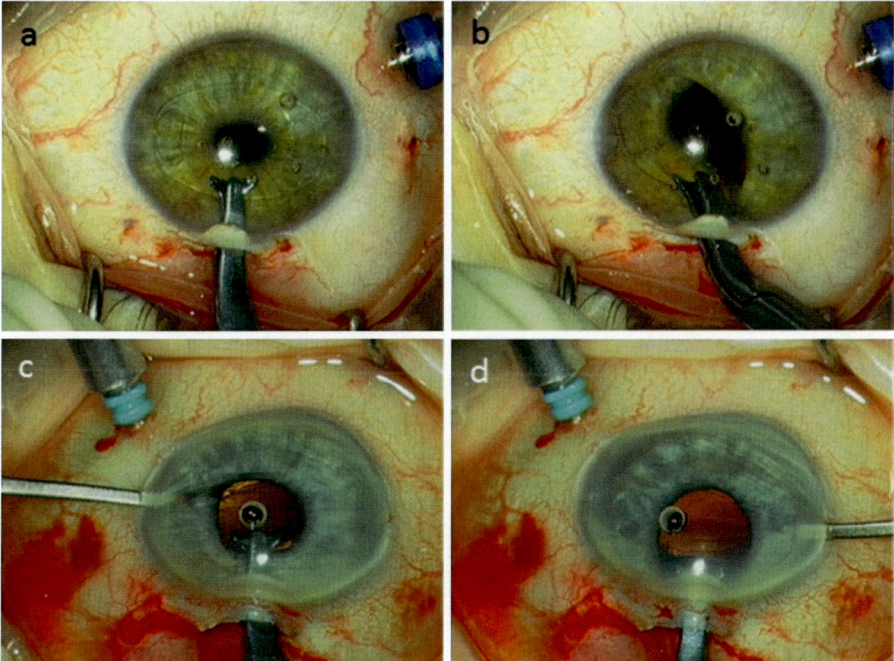

Fig. 16.13 (**a**) Centrate the IOL and fixate it with the IOL implantation forceps (AMO). (**b**) Tilt the IOL behind the iris on one side. (**c**) Tilt the IOL behind the iris on the other side and then press the iris tissue with the Sekundo enclavation spatula (Geuder) (no Sinskey hook instrument) behind the claws. (**d**) Switch hands and perform the same maneuver on the other side.

Fig. 16.14 Note the enclavated iris tissue at 3 and 9 o'clock

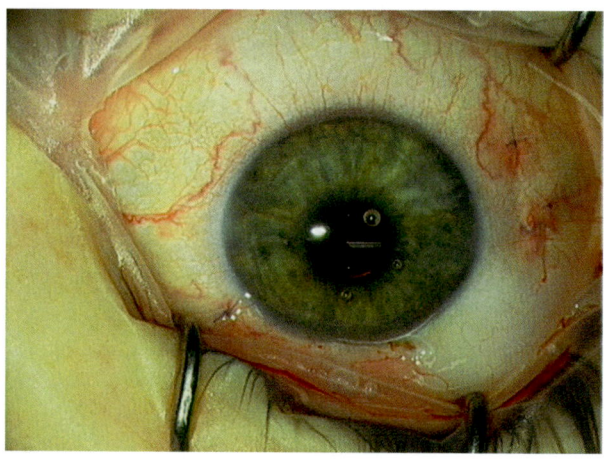

9. Closure of the frown incision and conjunctiva.

Suture the frown incision with a Vicryl 8–0 cross stitch and the conjunctiva with a Vicryl 8–0 interrupted stitch (Fig. 16.14).

Postoperative Treatment Combined Dexamethasone-Gentamicin drops 3x daily for 3 weeks. No mydriatics. If you want to do a dilated fundus exam later, it is absolutely safe to dilate with a iris claw IOL in place.

Complications

The Videos 16.4 and 16.6 demonstrate the surgical management of dislocated Artisan IOL.

Complete Iris-Claw IOL Dislocation The complete dislocation of an iris-claw IOL is very unusual. It may happen postoperatively secondary to a trauma. *See video*: Completely luxated iris-claw IOL after retropupillar fixation: https://www.youtube.com/watch?v=DrT9qPOxHac&list=PL0dKYclPD7yNZ1AT_ExbZazlu1UVppd-n&index=4

Partial Dislocation of an Iris-Claw IOL Perform a corneal 2,4 mm main incision. Elevate the IOL up pars plana and place the dislocated part of the IOL onto the iris and then fixate the loose side.

See video: An easy technique to reposition a luxated Artisan (Verisyse) IOL: https://www.youtube.com/watch?v=FhguhNRBPQY&t=117s

Postoperative inflammation due to traumatic surgery, which occurs only in the learning phase. Do not enclavate too much iris tissue. It may cause ocular pain. In order to avoid this side effect, use the thin enclavation spatula by Sekundo from Geuder.

FAQ

Is an iris-claw implantation after trauma possible?

If the eye underwent a traumatic surgery due to a difficult cataract surgery with loss of the lens capsule, we would prefer a delayed implantation. We would implant the iris claw IOL after approximately 1 month in order to obtain an uninflamed iris.

Why do you implant the Artisan IOL upside down?

The design of the Artisan IOL is convex; the haptics bend downwards. This makes them difficult to enclavate into the iris tissue. If you implant the Artisan IOL upside down, then the haptics are bent upwards and the enclavation is much easier.

Is an iridectomy necessary?

No, not in case of an upside-down implantation.

Yes, in case of a non-upside down implantation. Why? Because the IOL with the haptics have a convex shape. If you enclavate the IOL non-upside down then a pupillary block will occur. In the upside down position, however, the IOL has a concave shape preventing a pupillary block.

Is a core vitrectomy necessary?

A core vitrectomy increases the risk of a pseudophacodonesis. We perform therefore only an anterior vitrectomy.

Pupil dilatation before surgery?

Only 1–2 drops tropicamide. Do not dilate maximally because you need a small pupil for implantation.

Is it possible to perform this surgery in two sessions?

Yes, of course. You may in one session extract the IOL and perform an anterior vitrectomy and then in a second session implant an Artisan IOL. The advantage of two sessions is that the pupil can be constricted preoperatively with pilocarpine and that you work with a non-inflamed iris.

I am a beginner, what is the best eye to start with?

An aphakic eye with small pupil and removed anterior vitreous.

How do you treat a macular edema secondary to pseudophakia?

With topical eye drops, by posterior subtenon triamcinolone injection or with intravitreal triamcinolone injection.

Is a treatment with Ozurdex possible?

No. The Ozurdex pellet will enter the anterior chamber and cause a corneal damage. An Ozurdex injection is contraindicated in eyes with aphakia and aphakic Verisyse IOL's.

Remark The surgical technique of scleral fixation is demonstrated in a later chapter of this book.

Chapter 17
Surgical Management of Vitreous Prolapse Secondary to Ocular Trauma

In case of an open globe perforation we use a stepwise approach. In the first step we suture the scleral or corneal wound, In the second step we perform a cataract surgery or vitrectomy. In case of a scleral wound behind pars plana (4 mm behind the limbus) the retina is likely incarcerated in the wound and a vitrectomy is required. In case of a limbal wound (between limbus and 4 mm behind limbus) a vitreous prolapse is likely and a vitrectomy may be required. In case of a corneal wound the nucleus is affected and a cataract surgery is required.

In case of a corneal perforation we use the following approach: We close the cornea with single interrupted and cross stitches. We do not perform a cataract surgery or vitrectomy. We usually do not perform I/A of a hyphema because the iris may be damaged through surgery. Then we examine the patient once per week. If the IOP and inflammation can be regulated with anti-inflammatory and antihypertensive medication we wait 4 weeks. Why so long? During this period the damaged anterior capsule becomes fibrotic. A rhexis is much easier to perform and the IOL can be implanted in the lens capsule. If you operate early the rhexis is difficult and you may have to implant the IOL into the sulcus. The most difficult part of the surgery is the rhexis. You may need a lens capsule scissors and a rhexis forceps. Try always to implant the IOL into the capsular bag.

In case of a vitreous prolapse, an anterior vitrectomy is necessary. A core vitrectomy is not required. The trocar cannulas are placed away from the scleral wound. If for example a limbal perforation from 11 to 1 o'clock is present then place the trocar cannulas at 3, 5, 7 and 9 o'clock (Figs. 17.1 and 17.2).

© Springer Nature Switzerland AG 2020
U. Spandau, *Trocar Surgery for Cataract Surgeons*,
https://doi.org/10.1007/978-3-030-36093-1_17

Fig. 17.1 A limbal perforation from 11 to 1 o'clock. The wound was sutured and 4 weeks later a vitrectomy is performed

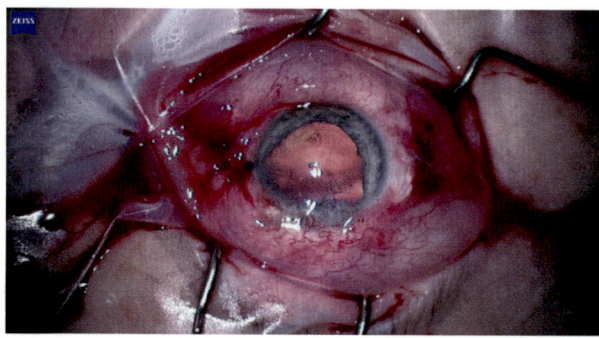

Fig. 17.2 Insert trocar cannulas away from the scleral wound. Good sites for trocar cannulas are 3, 5, 7 and 9 o'clock

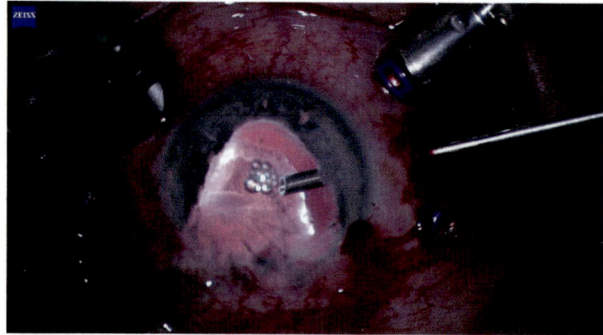

Part IV
Trocar Surgery of Posterior Segment

Chapter 18
Introduction and Possible Indications for Trocar Surgery of Posterior Segment

Trocar surgery of posterior segment with a phacoemulsification machine is possible for emergency cases such as dropped nucleus. This surgery has been performed successfully with the Catarex 3 (Oertli), Centurion (Alcon) and Infinity (Alcon).

18.1 Check List for Trocar Surgery of Posterior Segment

You want to operate a dropped nucleus or a posterior dislocated IOL. Are you confident with the following surgical steps you learned from trocar surgery of the anterior segment? See the following check list:

Trocar Surgery Techniques for Anterior Segment in a Stepwise Manner
1. Insertion and removal of 1 trocar on the temporal side
2. Anterior vitrectomy through trocar cannula
3. Master SICS
4. Elevation of anterior dislocated nucleus
5. Elevation of anterior dislocated IOL
6. Secondary IOL implantation
7. Insertion of two trocars on the temporal side; one trocar for irrigation line
8. Anterior vitrectomy from pars plana with infusion line

If you are acquainted to perform trocar surgery with two trocars, then you can proceed with the next steps:

Trocar Surgery Techniques for Posterior Segment in a Stepwise Manner
1. Insertion of three trocars
2. Usage of Biom and light fiber

Electronic Supplementary Material The online version of this chapter (https://doi. org/10.1007/978-3-030-36093-1_18) contains supplementary material, which is available to authorized users.

3. Core vitrectomy
4. Elevation of dropped nucleus
5. Elevation of dropped IOL

Start with insertion of three trocars, insertion of a light fiber and visualization of the retina (steps 1–2). If you can obtain a sharp picture of the retina, the next step will be the core vitrectomy (step 3). If you are acquainted with this step you can continue with the final steps which are elevation of a dropped nucleus and IOL (steps 4 and 5).

18.2   Possible Indications for Trocar Surgery of Posterior Segment

A dropped nucleus (Fig. 18.1) and a dropped IOL (Fig. 18.2) can be operated with a phacoemulsification machine. The modern phacoemulsification machines have novel anterior vitreous cutters with 23 Gauge. Before 20 Gauge was the standard for phacoemulsification machines. 23G trocars can be purchased from many companies (Alcon, Dorc, FCI, Mani). The companies Dorc (Netherlands), FCI (France) and Mani (Japan) offer sets with three trocars and one infusion line. Three trocars are inserted at pars plana, the infusion line is inserted in one trocar and the two other trocars are used for illumination and for the vitreous cutter (Figs. 18.3 and 18.4). The surgery of a vitrectomy is explained in detail in the final chapter of this book.

Fig. 18.1 Dropped nucleus

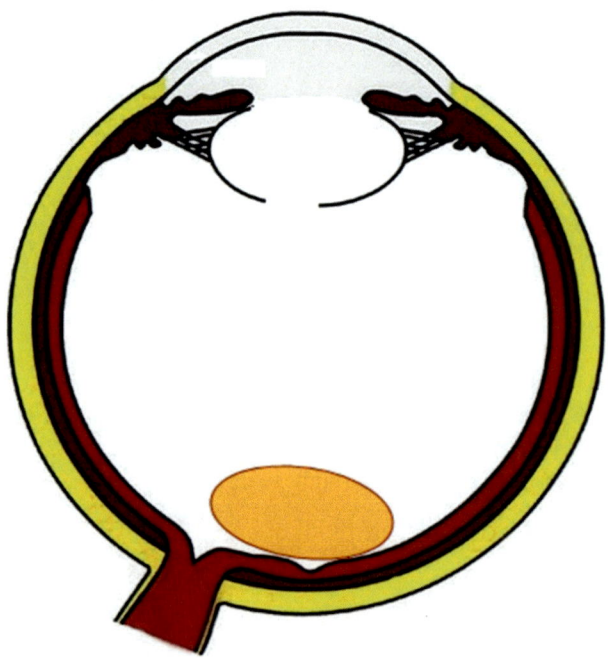

Fig. 18.2 Posterior dislocated IOL

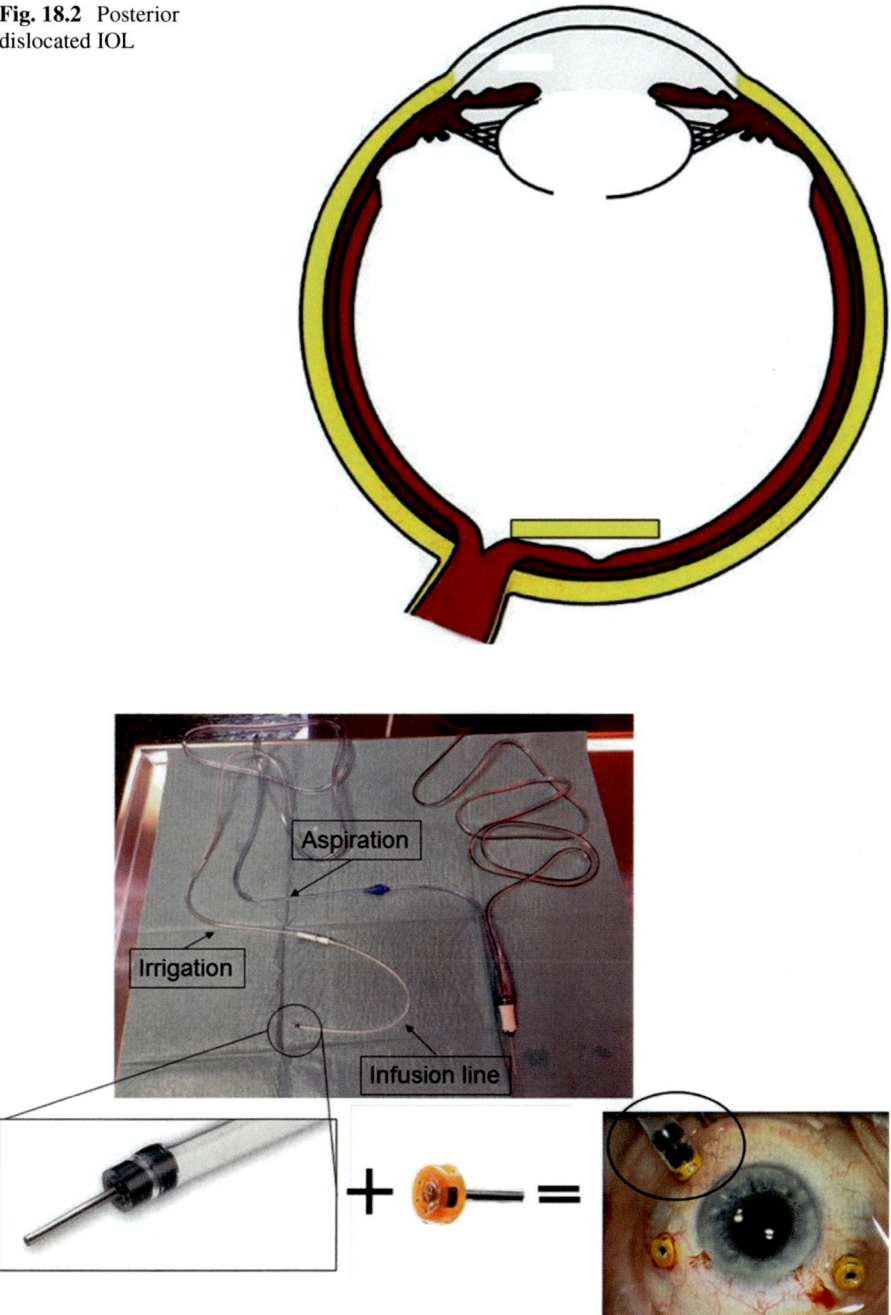

Fig. 18.3 Three 23G trocars are inserted. The irrigation from the cataract machine is connected to an infusion line (DORC, FCI, Mani) and inserted into the inferotemporal trocar

Fig. 18.4 The other two trocars are for the vitreous cutter and the light pipe. The vitreous cutter is a conventional anterior vitreous cutter and not a posterior segment vitreous cutter. The light pipe and the external light source must be purchased separately

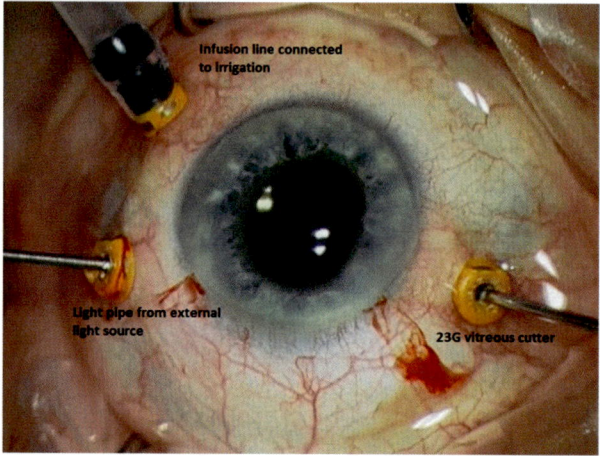

Fig. 18.5 Location designations in vitrectomy

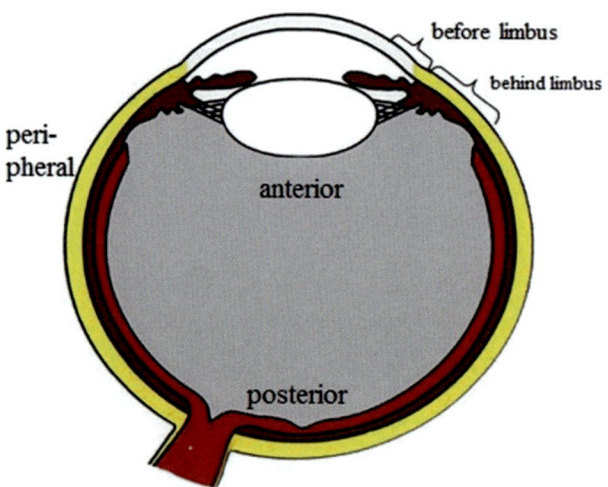

18.3   Anatomy of Pars Plana Vitrectomy

It is important to know the location designations of the eye during pars plana vitrectomy (Fig. 18.5). The lens is located anterior and the macula is located posterior. The trocar cannula is inserted behind the limbus. The pars plana is located between ciliary body and the peripheral retina (ora serrata).

18.4   Surgical Setup

The Video 18.1 demonstrates the surgical management of a pars plana vitrectomy with a cataract machine.

A vitrectomy with a cataract machine is possible. We perform combined vitrectomies and macular peeling for epiretinal membrane with an Infinity machine and a Centurion machine from Alcon (Fig. 18.5). Even combined phaco + vitrectomies are possible. We use the 23G vitreous cutters which are used for anterior vitrectomy. In addition, you need a viewing system and an illumination to visualize the retina. The viewing system is a BIOM (Oculus, Germany or RUV800, Leica, Germany) or a contact lens (Volk, USA). The illumination is a light fiber which is connected to an external light source (Photon, Synergetics).

Chapter 19
Equipment for Trocar Surgery of Posterior Segment

For posterior segment surgery the following devices and instruments are required:

1. Phacoemulsification machine
2. Viewing system
3. One 23G light fiber
4. One external light source
5. Anterior vitreous cutter (23G)
6. Three 23G trocars and 23G infusion line

19.1 Devices

Phacoemulsification Machines
All modern phacoemulsification machines can be employed for vitrectomy (Fig. 19.1). It is only important that the anterior vitreous cutter is available in 23 Gauge.

Settings for Posterior Segment
For settings we use continuous irrigation (Fig. 19.2). The irrigation pressure is different from machine to machine. It is approximately 35–40 mmHg for Centurion and 40–45 mmHg for Infinity. Look for a spontaneous retinal venous pulsation at the optic disc. For vitrectomy we use the setting I/A Cut.

Viewing System (Binocular Indirect Ophthalmo Microscope (BIOM System))
The optical quality of the surgical microscopes is excellent in all current models of the major manufacturers. More important is the viewing system. To obtain a sufficient view of the posterior segment, one needs either a plano-concave contact lens which is directly placed onto the cornea, or a highly refractive lens (60D, 90D, 120D) which is placed in front of the lens of the surgical microscope comparable to

© Springer Nature Switzerland AG 2020
U. Spandau, *Trocar Surgery for Cataract Surgeons*,
https://doi.org/10.1007/978-3-030-36093-1_19

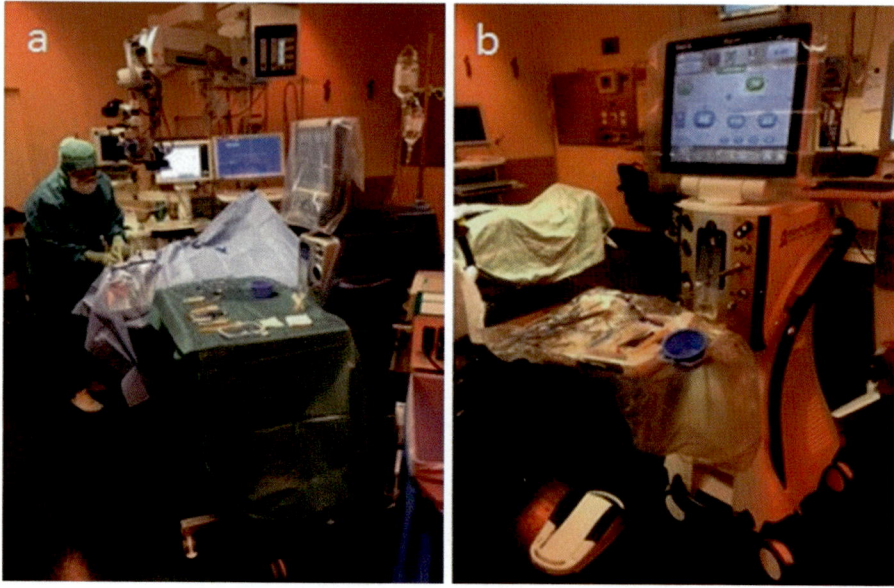

Fig. 19.1 (**a**) Vitrectomy with an Infinity machine (Alcon) and 23G cutter (2500 cpm). (**b**) Vitrectomy with a Centurion machine (Alcon) and 23G cutter (4000 cpm)

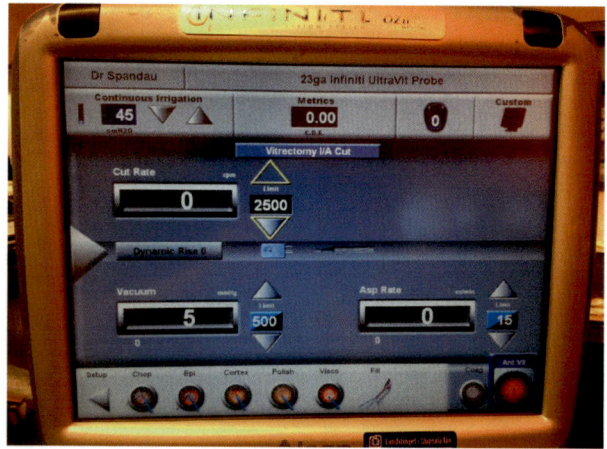

Fig. 19.2 Phaco settings for posterior vitrectomy with three trocars. Note Continuous irrigation. We use an Irrigation pressure of approximately 45 cmH$_2$O (= 33 mmHg). The vitrectomy setting is I/A Cut

indirect ophthalmoscopes. This results in an inverted image. By flicking a reversal system (so-called inverter) into the parallel beam path of the operating microscope an upright image is created.

The best viewing systems for high volume VR surgery are Resight from Zeiss, Germany and BIOM from Oculus, Germany. Both viewing systems require, however, an inverter. If you operate small volume VR surgery, then the Eibos (Möller-Wedel, Germany) or RUV800 (Leica, Germany) viewing system is a good option (Fig. 19.3). This viewing system is very easy to use, it requires no inverter and the view to fundus is excellent. For Eibos and RUV 800 no inverter is needed. The RUV800 system can only be used for Leica microscopes (Fig. 19.4).

Oculus (Germany) offers a one-way BIOM (Fig. 19.4) which is easy to use. The Oculus BIOM can be used with all microscopes. If you use a Zeiss microscope you have an option of attaching an inverterscope which is an eye piece having a built-in inverter which can be activated by a knob. The viewing system BIOM from Oculus provides a mirror image. Therefore, an *inverter* is installed in the microscope, which turns the mirror image of the BIOM. This must be turned on or off every time you switch between anterior segment or posterior segment view (by help of a knob or by a foot switch).

The company Oculus (Germany) has recently introduced a high-resolution lens with can be used as a 120D lens and at the same time as 60D peeling lens (Fig. 19.5).

Contact Lenses
Contact lens for retinal viewing can be for periphery (wide angle) and central use [1]. Both have direct and indirect types. Only indirect contact lens will require an inverter as their focal plane is close to the cornea and much away

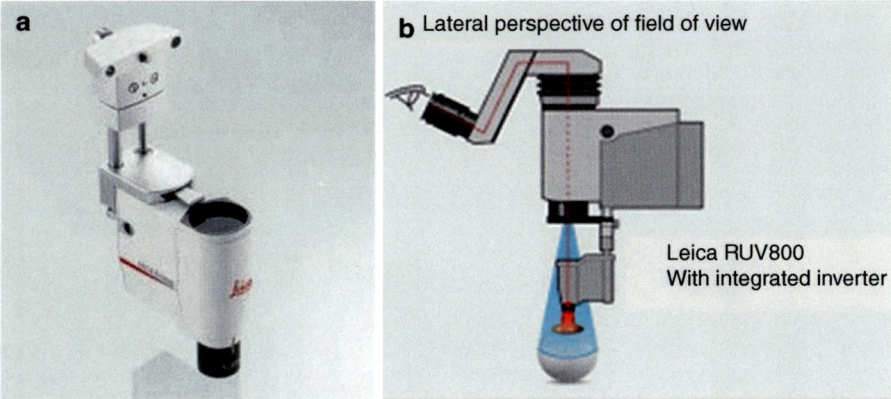

Fig. 19.3 RUV800 from Leica (**a**). The Leica viewing system has an integrated inverter (**b**)

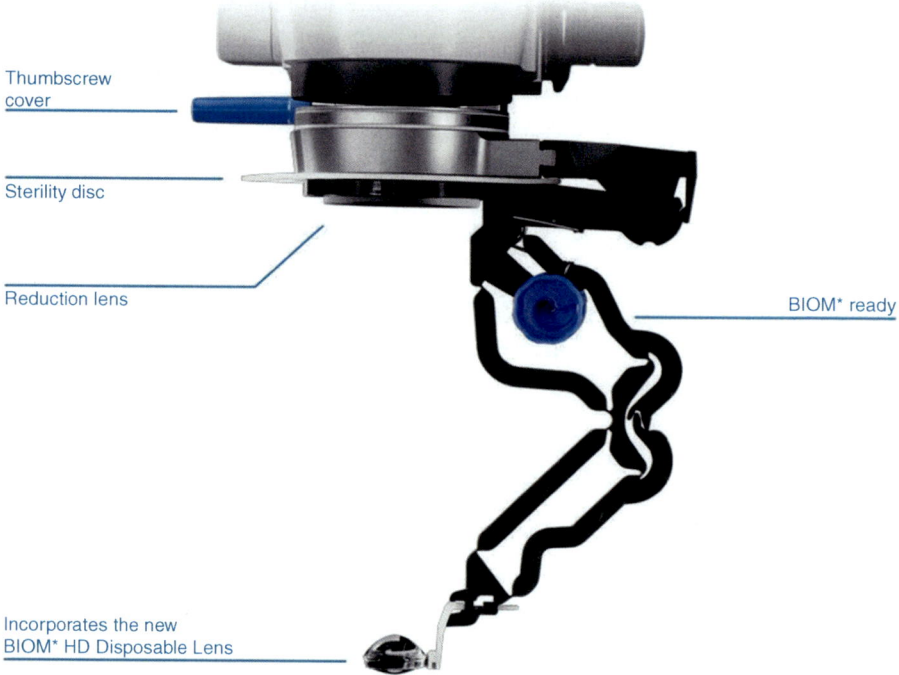

Thumbscrew
cover

Sterility disc

Reduction lens

BIOM* ready

Incorporates the new
BIOM* HD Disposable Lens

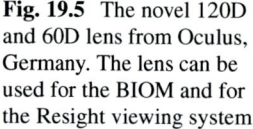

Fig. 19.4 A one-way BIOM from Oculus (Germany). Integrated is an inverter, which may be operated manually or by foot pedal. At the front of the BIOM the interchangeable front lenses are attached. https://www.oculussurgical.com/us/products/oculus-biom-ready/highlights/

Fig. 19.5 The novel 120D and 60D lens from Oculus, Germany. The lens can be used for the BIOM and for the Resight viewing system

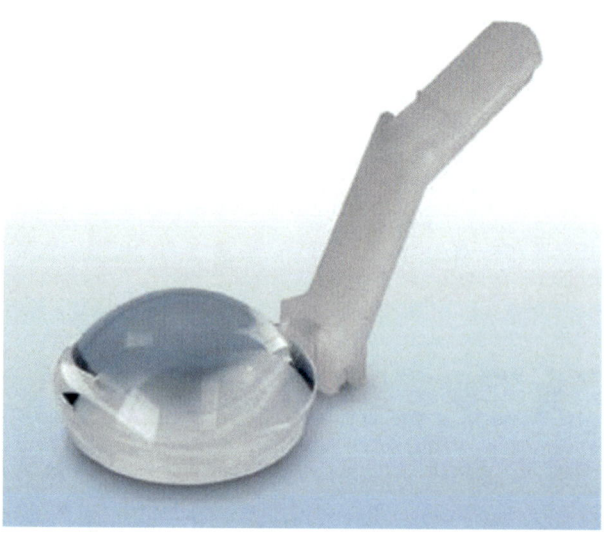

Fig. 19.6 Irrigating contact lens for viewing retina from Madhu Industries, Delhi (www. madhuinstruments.com)

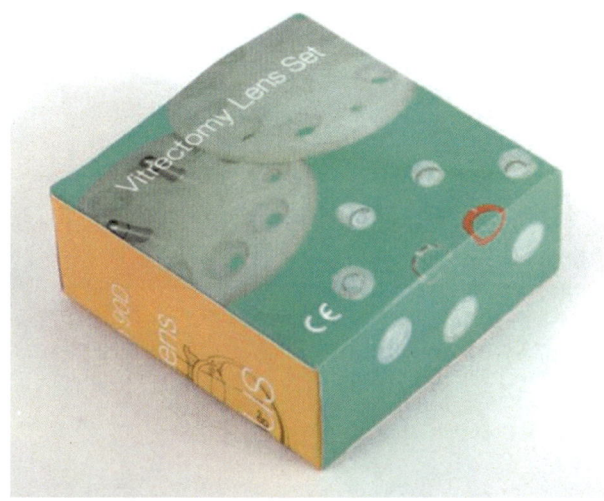

from the microscope objective lens. Regarding direct contact lenses for periphery work we can use Lander Lens 20°, 30° or 50° Tolentino prism (Ocular instruments). All these are also direct type, so no inverter needed (based on Landers design).

Indirect wide angle lens like HRX, MiniQuad XL from Volk also requires an inverter and used for a wide angle viewing. You can get similar design contact lens from Ocular instruments also. Remember: *Direct contact lens requires no inverter, indirect contact lens do need the inverter.*

Manufacturer: AVI, Grieshaber (Alcon), DORC, FCI Ophthalmics, Ocular instruments. Madhu Industries (Fig. 19.6). Aurolab does not manufacture contact lenses.

Conclusion

The RUV800 and Eibos viewing systems are robust and easy to use. They can only be used for Leica and Möller Wedel microscopes. A good alternative for all microscopes is the one-way viewing system BIOM from Oculus (Germany). This one-way BIOM has an excellent lens for peripheral view and for central fundus view.

A contact lens is a good and cheap alternative to a viewing system.

19.2   Instruments

The following instruments are required:

1. Three 23-gauge trocars (Figs. 19.7, 19.8, 19.9, 19.10)
2. 23-gauge infusion line (Fig. 19.11)

Fig. 19.7 23G One step cannula system from DORC No: 1272.ED206. This package includes three trocars and one infusion line

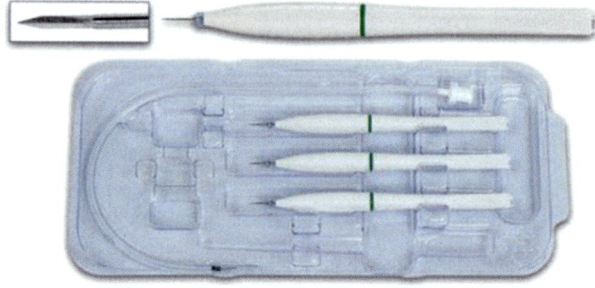

Fig. 19.8 This package includes three 23G trocars and one infusion line (FCI, France No. S9.7100.23)

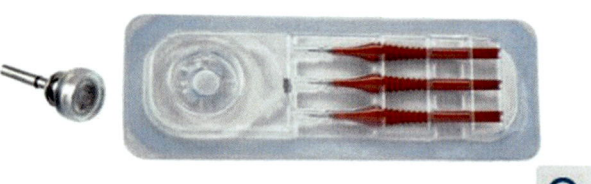

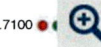

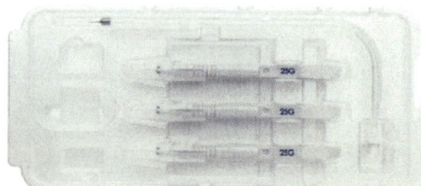

Product Name	Packaging	Order #
Trocar Kit 25G S	3 Kits / Box	MTK25S
Trocar Kit 23G S	3 Kits / Box	MTK23S

• Sterile 1 kit consists of 3 pcs. trocar with the valved cannula and 1 pc. infusion cannula.

Fig. 19.9 This package includes three 23G trocars and one infusion line (Mani, Japan MTK23S)

Fig. 19.10 This package includes three 23G trocars and one infusion line (Aurolab, India)

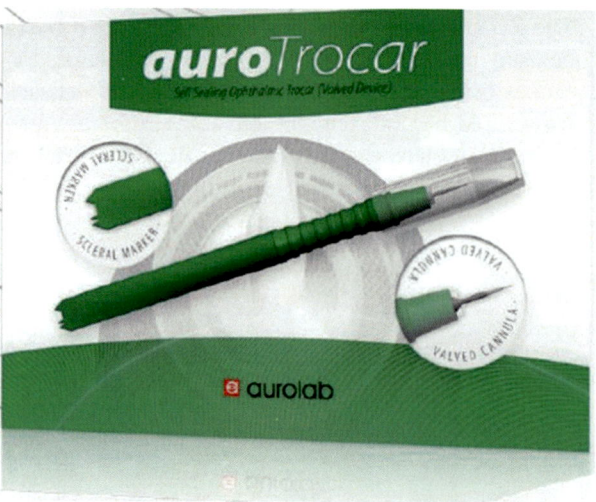

Fig. 19.11 Infusion line
(23G, DORC) No. 1279.
VFI. The infusion line can
be purchased separately
from DORC and Mani

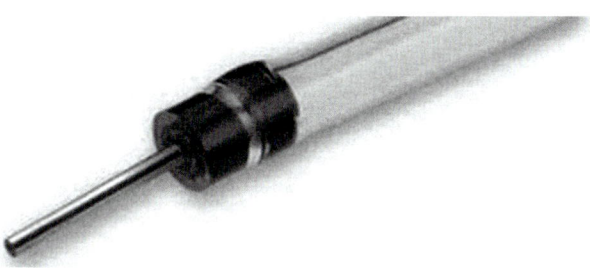

Fig. 19.12 An external
light source (Photon from
Synergetics, USA)
provides light for the light
pipe

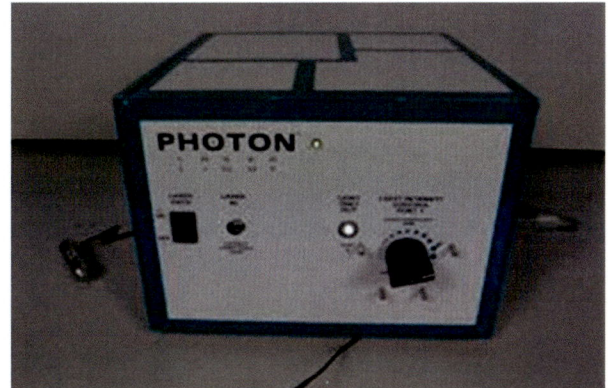

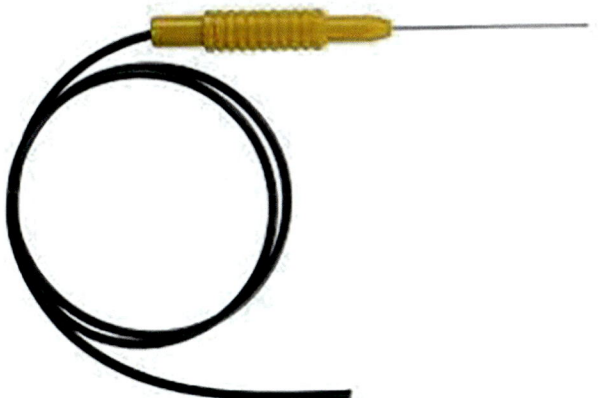

Fig. 19.13 Light pipe Synergetics (belongs to Bausch & Lomb) No. 56.21.23

The trocars and infusion line are available as a kit:

Illumination

For illumination an external light source (Fig. 19.12) and a light fiber (Fig. 19.13) is
required.

External Light Source

Conclusion: I am convinced that anterior and posterior segment surgery will fuse in the future. The modern cataract machines have a very powerful vitrectomy function today and employ 23G anterior vitreous cutters. In case of a dropped nucleus the cataract surgeon can convert with the same machine to a vitrectomy and remove the nuclear fragments.

Reference

1. Kakarla V, Chalam MD, Vinay A, Shah MD. Optics of wide-angle panoramic viewing system–assisted vitreous surgery. Surv Ophthalmol. 2004;49:437–45.

Chapter 20
Surgical Management of a Dropping and Dropped Nucleus

The surgical management of a dropped nucleus is usually in the hands of VR surgeons because a vitrectomy machine is required. But the new generation of phacoemulsification machines has a powerful vitreous cutter with good fluidics. A dropped nucleus surgery can be performed with these machines. There are three techniques for removal of the nucleus. (1) vitreous cutter, (2) elevation with PFCL and removal with SICS and (3) phacoemulsification. A vitreous cutter can be used if the nucleus is soft. If the nucleus is hard, I recommend an elevation of the nucleus into the anterior chamber with PFCL and the extraction with SICS technique. An alternative to the latter technique is an intravitreal phacoemulsification. For this technique we use a phacoemulsification machine and a regular phacoemulsification handpiece. The surgical technique is described in Sect. 20.5.

20.1 Recovery of a Dropping Nucleus from Pars Plana

The Videos 20.2 and 20.3 demonstrate the surgical management of a dropping nucleus from pars plana.

You must master this technique to become a complete cataract surgeon: To save a dropping nucleus and elevate it into the anterior chamber. A dropping nucleus can only be saved from pars plana and not from the anterior chamber because you need to place the viscoelastic cannula behind the nucleus (Fig. 20.1). You have to work fast otherwise the nucleus will be lost. If you suspect a dropping nucleus in an early stage of the surgery (e.g. large zonular lysis) then perform the sclerotomy or insert a trocar in advance in order to be prepared and not to lose time when the nucleus drops.

Electronic Supplementary Material The online version of this chapter (https://doi. org/10.1007/978-3-030-36093-1_20) contains supplementary material, which is available to authorized users.

Fig. 20.1 Nucleus
elevation from pars plana.
In case of a posterior
capsular defect and
luxation of the nucleus
insert a trocar and inject
viscoelastics (Viscoat®)
posterior to the nucleus.
Elevate then the nucleus
with the viscoelastic
cannula into the anterior
chamber

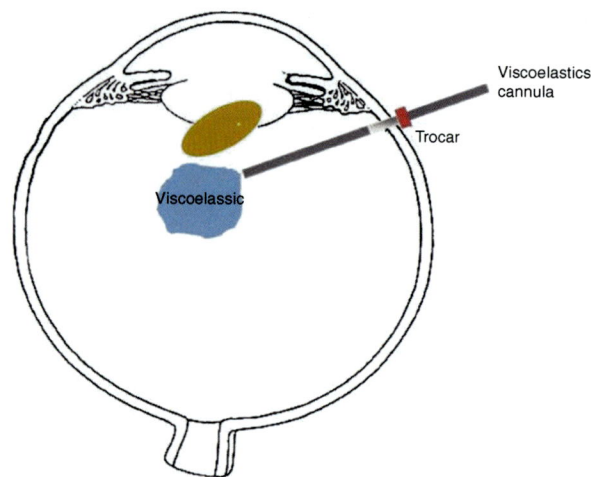

20.1.1   *Instrumentation*

1. Paracentesis knife e.g. 15° knife

   Or

2. 23G trocar

Stab the paracentesis knife 4 mm posterior the limbus into the middle of the eyeball (perpendicular); through the conjunctiva and the sclera. This manoeuvre is exactly the same as an intravitreal injection. Insert the viscoelastic cannula through the sclerotomy, place it behind the posterior capsule and inject viscoelastic behind the nucleus. Then elevate the nucleus with the viscoelastic cannula into the anterior chamber (Fig. 20.1).

Alternatively to a sclerotomy, you can insert a trocar (Fig. 20.1). The insertion of a trocar is fast, and the trocar has a distance marker for the sclerotomy. The viscoelastic cannula fits easily through the trocar.

The next steps are removal of the nucleus, anterior vitrectomy and secondary IOL implantation. For further details see also chapter "Posterior capsule rupture".

Tips and Tricks
The fastest method for retrieving of dropping nucleus: Attach a 27G needle cannula to the viscoelastic syringe (such as in Fig. 20.1), pierce the needle through the sclera (3,5 mm behind the limbus) and inject viscoelastic behind the nucleus.

20.2   Operative Planning and Strategies for Surgical Management of Dropped Nucleus

The Videos 20.1, 20.2, 20.3, and 20.4 demonstrate the surgical management of a dropped nucleus with a phacoemulsification machine:

Removal of Dropped Nucleus A soft nucleus and cortex can be removed with a vitreous cutter. A hard nucleus can only be removed with a fragmatome. A fragmatome is a phacoemulsification handpiece without sleeve. It is used without trocar cannula. The fragmatome is inserted through a 20G sclerotomy without trocar cannula. A fragmatome *cannot* be used with a cataract machine. You can use instead a phacoemulsification handpiece without sleeve. The phaco needle is shorter than a fragmatome needle.

Necessity of Surgery If nuclear fragments drop, we always operate in order to prevent intraocular inflammation and hypertension. In case of dropped soft cortical fragments, it is possible to wait and delay surgery as long as the eye remains quiet.

Timing of Surgery The surgery is not an emergency. Normally a dropped nucleus occurs under topical anesthesia. To proceed with vitrectomy under drop anesthesia will inflict much unnecessary pain to the patient. It is therefore advisable to stop surgery when a dropped nucleus occurs and to schedule a planned surgery within 1 week. During this time the eye must be treated for inflammation and ocular hypertension so that the cornea is clear for the surgery.

Tips and Tricks
The most patients who underwent a *complicated cataract surgery* do not complain about the complication but about the painful procedure. Why? The cataract surgery was performed with topical anesthesia and when the complication occurred the surgery was continued with the same anesthesia. Our recommendation: If you experience a complication, decide if you continue or stop the surgery. If you decide to continue then add a subtenon or retrobulbar anesthesia. I recommend the injection of 3 cc Carbocaine (Mepivacaine) into the caruncle. You will have a happy patient and an easy surgery.

The most difficult part of this surgery is the removal of the nucleus. There are two methods (Fig. 20.2).

1. Epinucleus and soft nuclear fragments can be removed with the vitreous cutter. But hard and big nuclear fragments *cannot* be removed with the vitreous cutter. In this case the following method must be applied.
2. After vitrectomy, you can elevate the nucleus with PFCL to the pupillary plane and remove it there with a conventional phaco hand piece or the SICS technique. The latter technique is very elegant and easy in case of a rock-hard nucleus. For details of SICS technique see this book "Part III: General surgical techniques".

Surgical planning: Two things should be assessed preoperatively:

1. How much of the nucleus is luxated? Is it a soft or hard nucleus? Or did only cortical fragments drop? In case of a complete nucleus drop I recommend removal with PFCL and SICS technique. In case of a soft nucleus I recommend to remove it with a vitreous cutter. In case of a hard fragment I recommend a phacoemulsification handpiece.

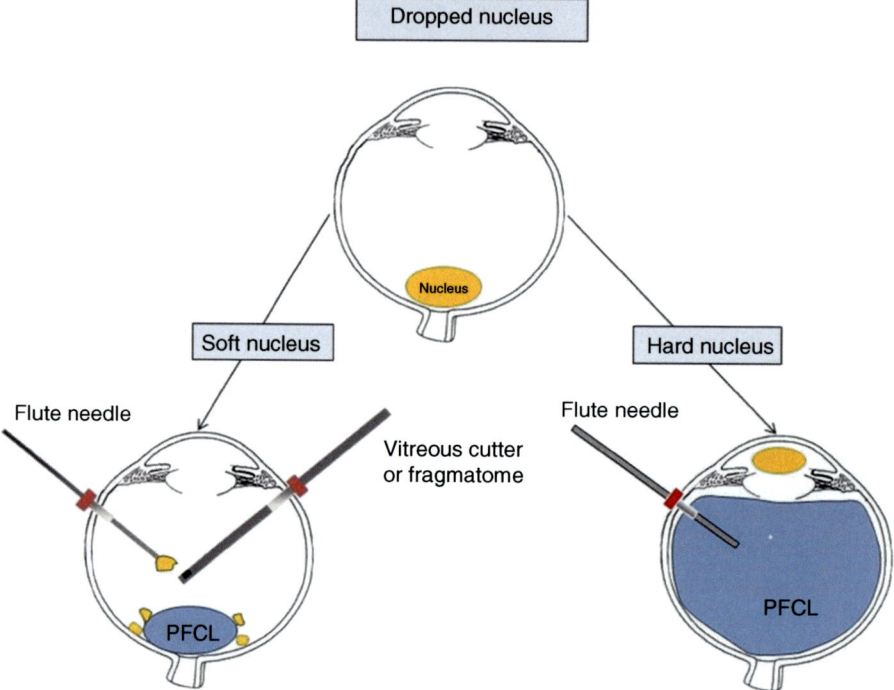

Fig. 20.2   Treatment algorithm for removal of soft or hard dropped nucleus

2. Assess preoperatively whether the anterior capsule is intact. If the anterior capsule is intact, implant a three-piece IOL in the sulcus. If it is not intact, you can implant a scleral fixated or even easier an iris fixated IOL.

20.3   Extraction of a Posteriorly Dislocated Nucleus with Vitreous Cutter

The limitation of a dropped nucleus removal with the phacoemulsification machine is that a fragmatome cannot be used. Do you know which tissue you can remove with a vitreous cutter? This is an important knowledge for this case. With the vitreous cutter, you can remove cortex, epinucleus, a soft nucleus and iris tissue. You cannot remove a hard nucleus or a thick capsular fibrosis. To remove a hard nucleus, it is advisable to perform phaco at the pupillary plane or a SICS.

The Videos 20.1, 20.2, 20.3, and 20.4 demonstrate the surgical management of a dropped nucleus with a PFCL.

Instruments
1. 23G trocars and infusion line
2. Illumination: Chandelier light fiber or hand-held light fiber

3. Viewing system
4. Anterior vitreous cutter

Individual Steps
1. 23G 3-port system with chandelier light fiber
2. Anterior vitrectomy via pars plana
3. Removal of residual cortex from the lens capsule via paracentesis
4. Core vitrectomy, if necessary PVD
5. PFCL for macula protection.
6. Removal of nuclear fragments with vitreous cutter and flute needle
7. Vitrectomy of peripheral vitreous
8. Implantation of an intraocular lens
9. Removal of trocar cannulas

The Surgery Step-by-Step: (Figs. 20.3, 20.4, 20.5, and 20.6)
1. 3-port system with chandelier light fiber

After insertion of three trocars we insert a chandelier light fiber, because we work bimanually in step 6.

2. Anterior vitrectomy via pars plana
3. Removal of residual cortex from the lens capsule via paracentesis
4. Core vitrectomy, if necessary PVD

The anterior vitreous is removed with the vitreous cutter via pars plana (Fig. 20.3). Make circular movements with the vitreous cutter. The vitreous cutter port points towards the posterior pole in order to avoid a damage of the lens capsule. Aspirate then the residual cortex with the vitreous cutter via a paracentesis. If vitreous clogs the port of the vitreous cutter during aspiration, then cut vitreous first. Alternatively, you can use two I/A hand pieces. It is important that you switch the vitreous cutter to aspiration and not to cutting; otherwise you risk destroying the anterior capsule.

If the lens capsule is free from cortex, continue with a core vitrectomy from pars plana. There are two possible scenarios regarding the vitreous. The posterior vitreous may be *detached* (PVD) (see Fig. 20.4) or the posterior vitreous may be

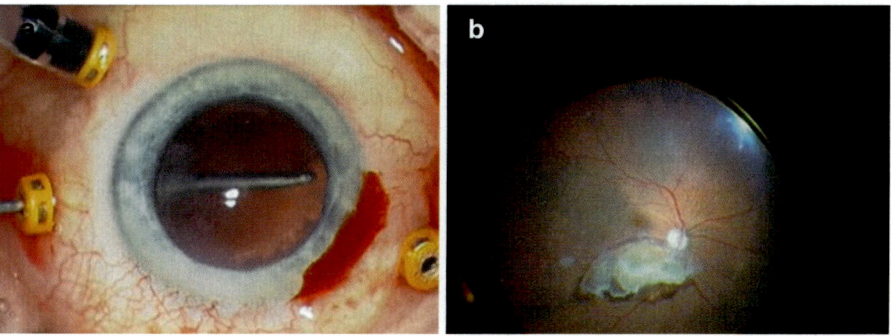

Fig. 20.3 (**a**) Anterior vitrectomy from pars plana in an eye with PCR. (**b**) Dropped nucleus

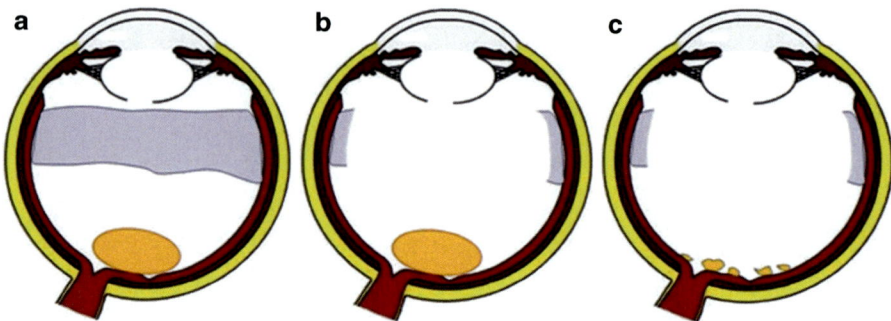

Fig. 20.4 (**a**) The posterior vitreous is *detached*. (**b**) After removal of the central vitreous. (**c**) The nuclear fragments have no contact with the vitreous

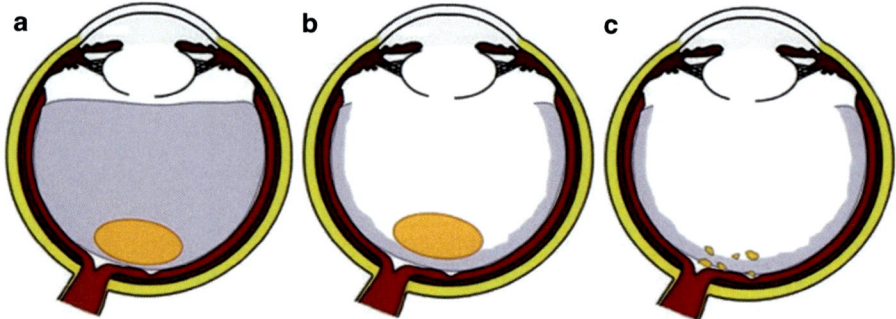

Fig. 20.5 (**a**) The posterior vitreous is *attached*. (**b**) After removal of the central vitreous. The posterior vitreous is still attached and present. (**c**) Some nuclear fragments are located above the vitreous and easy to remove. But some nuclear fragments are localized behind the vitreous which are difficult to remove because the vitreous is in the way

attached (no PVD) (see Fig. 20.5). If a PVD is present, then you remove the anterior and central vitreous (Fig. 20.4b). The nucleus is located on the retina and has no contact with the vitreous (Fig. 20.4c). If a PVD is absent, then you remove the anterior and central vitreous but not the posterior vitreous (Fig. 20.5b). The nucleus is, therefore, in contact with the vitreous (Fig. 20.5b). After removal of the large nucleus small nuclear fragments remain. They may be located above the vitreous or behind the vitreous (Fig. 20.5c). Those fragments which are located behind the vitreous are difficult to extract because the vitreous is in the way. In this case a posterior vitreous detachment must be performed.

5. PFCL for macula protection
6. Removal of nuclear fragments with vitreous cutter and flute needle

Inject next a small PFCL bubble to protect the macula. Soft lens material can be removed easily with the vitreous cutter. Thick lens material is removed best bimanual with flute needle and vitreous cutter. Aspirate the lens fragments with the flute needle, move the needle to the central vitreous cavity and remove them

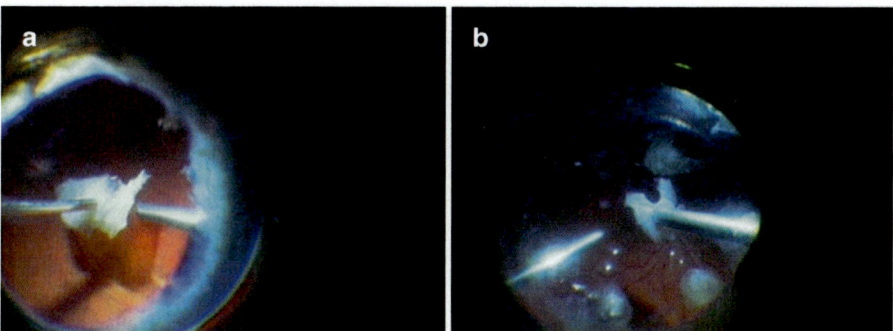

Fig. 20.6 Bimanual surgery. (**a**) Many small nuclear fragments. Every fragment has to be removed. (**b**) The left hand fixates the fragment with a flute needle (backflush instrument) and the right hand removes it with the vitreous cutter

there safely with the vitreous cutter. Then crush the nucleus with the flute needle. This procedure is performed repeatedly until all the lens fragments are removed (Fig. 20.6).

If you perform this procedure without flute needle (only with the vitreous cutter), there is a risk that during the frequent aspiration of the lens fragments with the vitreous cutter you may injure the retina (retinal break) or the choroid (choroidal hemorrhage). In addition, the frequent aspiration of the lens fragments clogs the vitreous cutter and the flute needle. It is advisable that the scrub nurse repeatedly cleans both instruments from nuclear fragments. If the suction is not working properly, the risk is increased to induce damage to the retina or choroid. In this case, it is advisable to inject a PFCL bubble in order to elevate the nucleus and protect the posterior pole.

7. Vitrectomy of peripheral vitreous

The vitreous cutter breaks the nucleus in many small pieces which are dispersed all over the posterior segment. These fragments must be removed meticulously, because every nucleus fragment which remains may cause a postoperative sterile uveitis. The most lens fragments are located in the vitreous base at 6 o'clock. In order to visualize and remove them you need to self indent the vitreous with the scleral depressor. For this procedure use a chandelier light.

Tips and Tricks
The trimming of the vitreous base is an important step because a *residual nuclear fragment* will cause a postoperative sterile uveitis. Check the periphery 360 degrees and particularly at 6 o'clock. Conclusion: Do not be satisfied after removal of the big fragments but after complete removal of all small fragments.

8. Implantation of the IOL
9. Removal of trocar cannulas

If the anterior capsule is intact, the lens can be implanted into the sulcus with optic capture inside the anterior capsulorhexis. If not, fixate a 3-piece IOL to the sclera or implant an iris-fixated IOL (Artisan®, Verisyse®).

Tips and Tricks
1-piece IOL vs 3-piece IOL: Do not implant a 1-piece IOL into the sulcus because the haptics cause a focal depigmentation of the iris resulting in a secondary pigment glaucoma (iris chaffing). This does not happen with a 3-piece IOL. The reason for this is that a 1-piece IOL has thick and sharp haptics whereas 3-piece haptics are round and thin

Postoperative Treatment for Conventional Vitrectomy: Combined Dexamethasone-Gentamicin drops 5× daily for 2 weeks and 3× daily for third week. Atropine drops 1× daily for 2 weeks.

20.4 Extraction of a Posteriorly Dislocated Nucleus (Dropped Nucleus) with PFCL

With this technique, the nucleus is luxated with PFCL into the anterior chamber and removed with a SICS technique or with phacoemulsification. The advantages of a SICS technique are a fast and complete removal of the dropped nucleus. The disadvantage is sometimes a damage of the anterior lens capsule when luxating the nucleus into the anterior chamber. The advantage of phacoemulsification is that we are more used to this technique. The disadvantage is an injury of the endothelium because the phacoemulsification is performed in the anterior chamber.

The Video 20.5 demonstrate the surgical management of a dropped nucleus with a phacoemulsification machine.

Instruments
1. 3-port trocar system with chandelier light
2. Crescent angled bevel up knife
3. Tunnel knife, 2.4 mm
4. Double-barrelled (dual bore) infusion cannula (Fig. 20.7)

Tamponade
Intraoperative: PFCL
    Postoperative: None

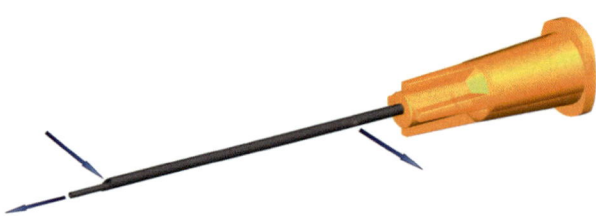

Fig. 20.7 Double-barreled (dual bore) cannula. This cannula is used for the injection of fluids. This special cannula injects PFCL into the eye and at the same time allows egress of fluid from the eye passively. The cannula prevents an intraocular hypertension during injection. The injection is done monomanual, a chandelier light is not required. DORC: Double bore cannula. EFD.06

Individual Step
1. 3-port trocar system with chandelier light.
2. Vitrectomy.
3. Injection of PFCL and elavation of the nucleus to the pupillary plane.
4. Phacoemulsification of the nucleus.

   OR

5. Extraction of the nucleus with the SICS method.
6. Implantation of an intraocular lens.
7. Removal of trocars.

The Surgery Step-by-Step (Figs. 20.8, 20.9, 20.10, and 20.11)
1. 3-port trocar system with chandelier light
2. Vitrectomy
3. Injection of PFCL and elevation of the nucleus to the pupillary plane

The anterior vitreous is removed with the vitreous cutter via pars plana. Then the residual cortex is aspirated from the lens capsule with the vitreous cutter via a paracentesis. It is important that you switch the vitreous cutter to aspiration and not to cutting. Otherwise there is a risk of injuring the anterior capsule. If the lens capsule is free from the cortex, continue with vitrectomy from pars plana.

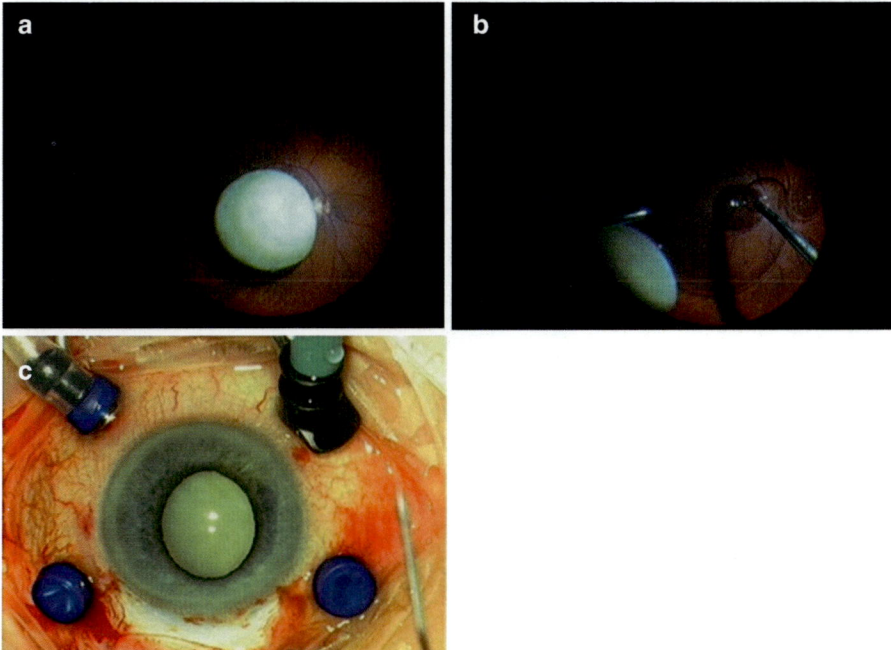

Fig. 20.8 (**a**) A luxated white nucleus secondary to trauma which happened 20 years ago. (**b**) PFCL (heavy liquid) is injected to elevate the nucleus. (**c**) The nucleus is now located behind the pupil

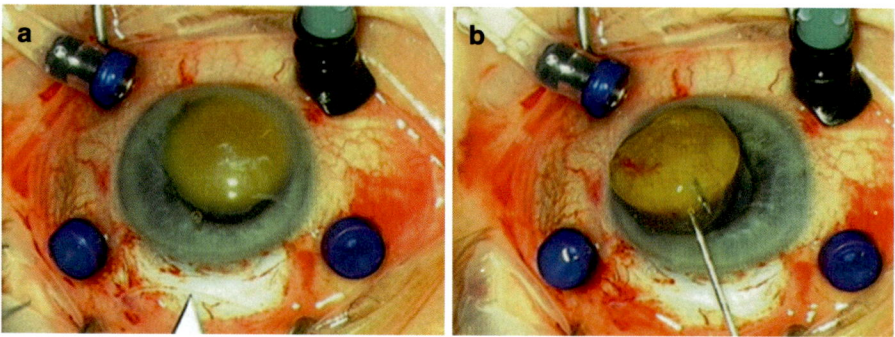

Fig. 20.9 (**a**) Then the nucleus is luxated into the anterior chamber. This maneuver is not so easy because the lens capsule is slippery. Now an 8 mm frown incision is performed. (**b**) The nucleus is removed with a so-called fish hook. Use alternatively a serrated lens loop.

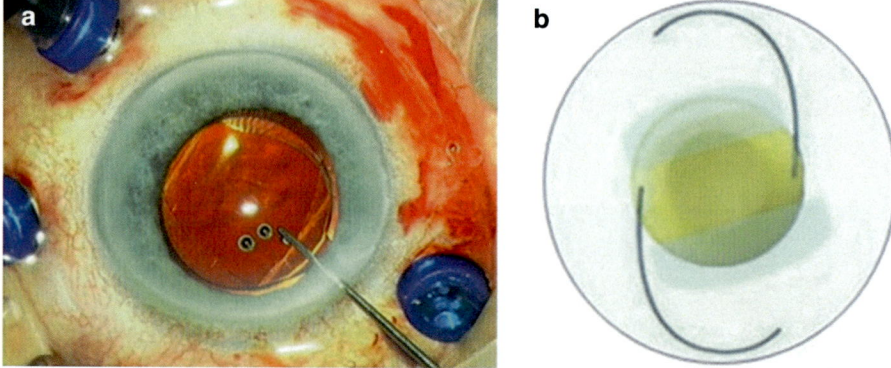

Fig. 20.10 (**a**) Insert a 3-piece IOL with haptics in the sulcus and the optic behind the rhexis (**b**) An illustration of "haptic out, optic in". The IOL is centrated and a barrier between posterior and anterior segment is created

Fig. 20.11 If the lens capsule is absent then implant scleral fixated IOL or iris fixated IOL (Artisan (Opthec, Netherlands), Verisyse (AMO, USA))

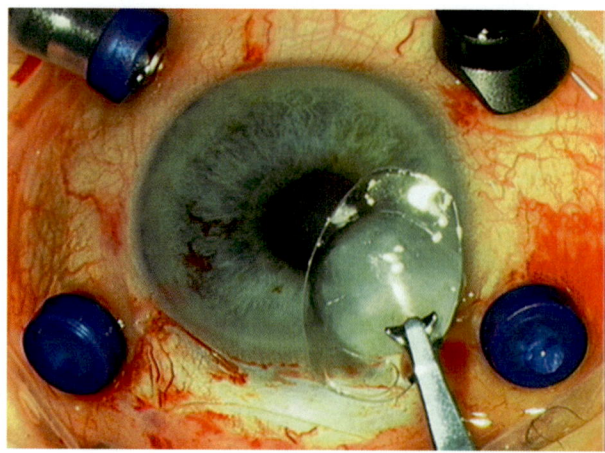

Instill a PFCL bubble with the dual bore cannula. This can be done monomanual. If necessary, lift up the nucleus with the flute instrument onto the PFCL bubble (Fig. 20.8). Then inject PFCL up to the sclerotomies; the nucleus is then slowly elevated up to the level of the pupil (Fig. 20.8c).

Tips and Tricks
Dropped nucleus: The difficulty of this step is that the nucleus is located on the posterior pole so that a damage of the retina is easily induced. Three advices: (1) Inject a PFCL bubble to (a) protect the macula and (b) elevate the nucleus. (2) Work bimanual so that one hand can fixate the nucleus and the other hand can remove it. (3) If the posterior vitreous is attached, then the vitreous cortex is like a cushion for the nucleus making its removal difficult, in this case induce a PVD to free the access to the nucleus. For details see chapter "pars plana vitrectomy step-by-step".

4. Phacoemulsification of the nucleus

Emulsify next the nucleus with a normal phaco hand piece. The phacoemulsification disintegrates the nucleus into small pieces which may slide away on the PFCL bubble in the retinal periphery and must be retrieved from there. Viscoelastics (Viscoat®) behind the nucleus can help to hold the lens fragments in the pupil. It may, however, be advisable to emulsify the nucleus in the anterior chamber. A phacoemulsification in the anterior chamber may, however, cause a significant endothelial cell loss. *Remark*: Use repeated viscoat if you want to emulsify nucleus in anterior chamber
OR

5. Extraction of the nucleus with the SICS method

If the nucleus is too hard for the phaco, you can extract the nucleus faster and with a lower risk of complications in toto (Fig. 20.9). I recommend the so-called SICS technique (small incision cataract surgery), which is a modified form of ECCE. In short: limbal peritomy from 11 to 1 o'clock with Vannas scissors, mark then with the caliper a 9-mm wide frown incision, dissect the frown incision and a scleral tunnel with a crescent bevel up knife, open the anterior chamber with a 2.4 mm tunnel knife. The next steps are the luxation of the nucleus into the anterior chamber, injection of viscoelastics (Viscoat®) below and above the nucleus and finally extraction of the nucleus with a serrated lens loop, fish hook or viscoelastics. The incision may be sutured with a Vicryl 8–0 cross stitch.

6. Implantation of the intraocular lens
7. Removal of trocars

If the anterior capsule is intact, the lens is implanted into the sulcus ("haptic out, optic in") (Fig. 20.10). If not, fixate a lens to the sclera or to the iris (e.g., iris fixated IOL) (Fig. 20.11).

Complications
If you remove the nuclear fragments monomanually, then you risk damaging the retina and choroid. Retinal break and choroidal hemorrhage are the most common complications and can be avoided, when you work bimanually.

If you work bimanually with chandelier light, then you can hold in one hand the vitreous cutter and in the other hand a Charles flute needle. You can pick up the small fragments with the Charles flute needle and remove them safely in the middle of the vitreous cavity with the vitreous cutter.

FAQ

Which method do you prefer, SICS?

In case of a hard nucleus I prefer SICS because this technique is faster and smoother and removes the complete nucleus. In case of a medium hard nucleus I would prefer the phacoemulsification.

I dislike about the phacoemulsification technique that it breaks the nucleus in many small pieces. And all pieces must be meticulously removed. Only one remaining nuclear fragment can cause a sterile endophthalmitis. This problem does not exist with the SICS technique.

I have two problems: First, did you do PVD during removal of posterior lens fragments? I once suffered secondary retinal detachment after similar procedure. Second, I noticed that the central part anterior vitreous had been cleaned owed to triamcinolone acetonide, but when doing I/A behind iris, is there a possibility that traction is induced onto the peripheral anterior vitreous thus resulting into tiny holes? And how to avoid these problems?

A PVD is not necessary. But if a PVD is not present you may have the following problems: (1) If you use PFCL then small PFCL bubbles may hide behind the vitreous cortex and are difficult to remove. (2) Or small nuclear fragments may hide behind vitreous cortex and be difficult to remove.

I/A behind iris: If you remove cortex from the lens capsule with I/A you may aspirate vitreous and the vitreous traction may cause holes. To avoid this problem, start with an anterior vitrectomy from pars plana. This takes 3–5 min. Then continue with removal of cortex. You can do this with the vitreous cutter (but be careful) or with I/A. If you again aspirate vitreous then stop I/A and continue again with vitrectomy. Stain also always the vitreous with triamcinolone.

The complete surgery of dropped nucleus is presented as a drawing in Fig. 20.12.

20.5   Extraction of a Posteriorly Dislocated Nucleus with Intravitreal Phacoemulsification

The extraction of a dropped nucleus with an intravitreal phacoemulsification is not widely established yet. Ruiz Moreno and colleagues use a vitrectomy machine for dropped nucleus surgery but for intravitreal phacoemulsification they use a regular phacoemulsification handpiece (and not a fragmatome) as a routine [1]. They say that the phacoemulsification handpiece is better than

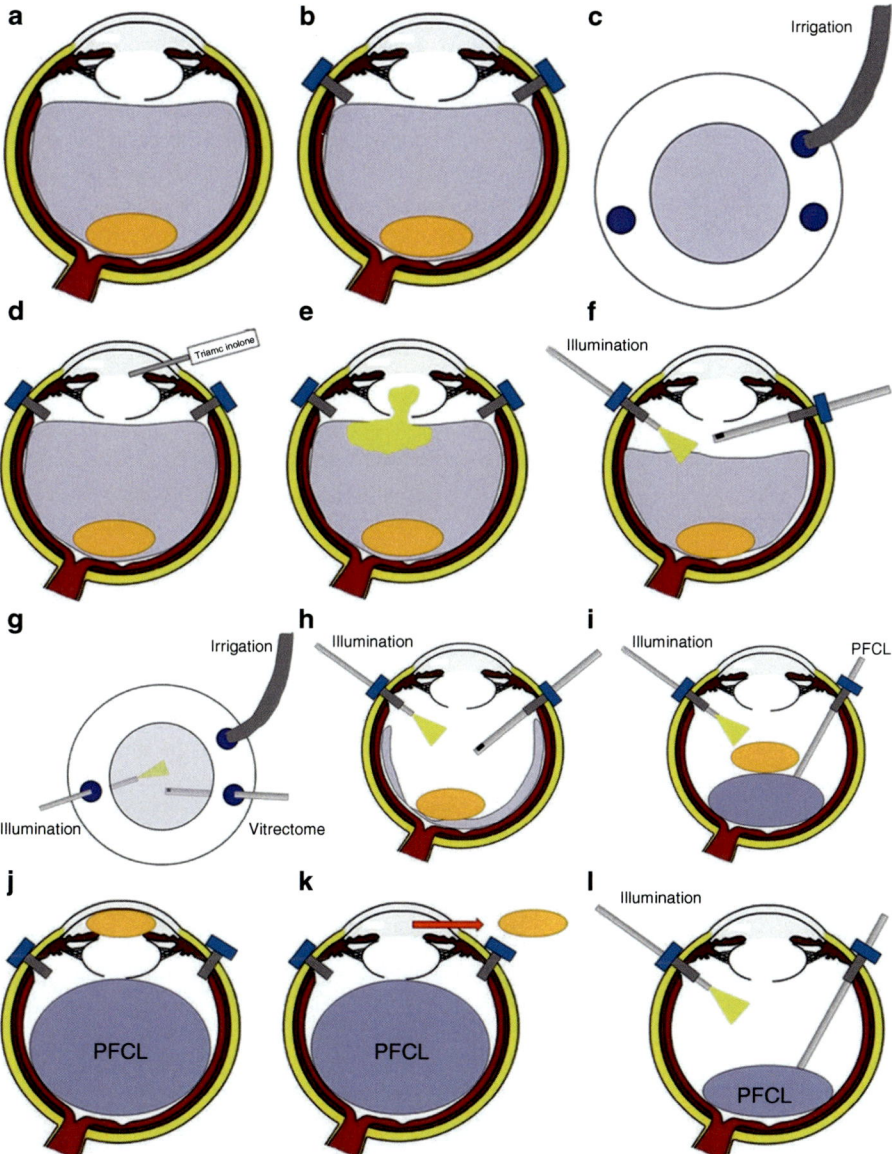

Fig. 20.12 The complete surgery of dropped nucleus at a glance. (**a**) Dropped nucleus, (**b**) insertion of three trocars, (**c**) insert infusion line, (**d**) inject triamcinolone, (**e**) the anterior vitreous is well stained, (**f**) removal of anterior vitreous, (**g, h**) vitrectomy with light fiber and anterior vitreous cutter, (**i**) injection of PFCL, (**j**) further injection of PFCL until the nucleus is elevated to the anterior chamber, (**k**) removal of the nucleus, (**l**) removal of PFCL with Charles flute needle

fragmatome because it is peristaltic and keeps lens fragments attached to the phacotip with less chattering. Ruiz Moreno uses a standard phaco needle with 50% phaco power and vacuum of only 100 mm Hg. They conclude that PPV with intravitreal phacoemulsification is the technique of choice for dislocated nuclei [1, 2, 3]. In this chapter I will demonstrate a complete dropped nucleus surgery only with a cataract machine (Infinity, Alcon). I will use an anterior vitreous cutter and a phacoemulsification handpiece.

The Video 20.6 demonstrates the extraction of a dropped nucleus with an Infinity machine and phacoemulsification handpiece.

- On you tube: This surgery was performed with a Catarex 3 from Oertli and a phaconeedle of 2.2 mm. https://www.youtube.com/watch?v=Qusvb8l7UJY&feature=youtu.be

Instruments

Fragmatome/phacoemulsificationhandpiece: A fragmatome and a phacoemulsification handpiece are identical except for different needles. The fragmatome needle is longer than the phaco needle. You can use a normal phacoemulsification handpiece with a normal phaco needle but without sleeve (Fig. 20.13). Remove the irrigation tube from the phaco handpiece. Only the aspiration tubing is connected to the phaco handpiece. The irrigation is placed via an irrigation line into a trocar cannula at pars plana. The phaco handpiece requires a 20G sclerotomy without trocar cannula. I recommend three trocar cannulas (one for irrigation line, one for light fiber and one for vitreous scutter) and one 20G sclerotomy without trocar cannula. The latter is located between the two temporal cannulas and is for the intravitreal phacoemulsification handpiece. For settings I recommend low aspiration or the sculpting mode.

A fragmatome or intravitreal phacoemulsification handpiece is difficult to use. On the one hand, the removal of a nucleus is more difficult inside the vitreous cavity than within the lens capsule. Lens fragments tend to jump away from the needle tip but this behaviour is more prominent in a fragmatome than a phacoemulsification handpiece. High levels of suction inside the vitreous cavity must be avoided. Aspiration of the vitreous or retinal damage may occur (retinal detachment or choroidal damage).

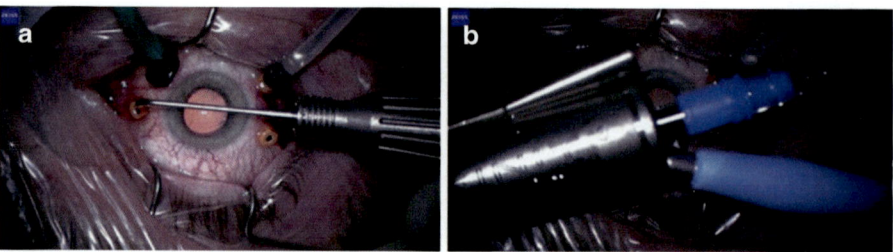

Fig. 20.13 (**a**) Remove the sleeve from the phaco needle. A regular needle is used. (**b**) Remove the irrigation tubing and attach the aspiration tubing

The dropped nucleus is removed with the vitreous cutter and the phacoemulsification handpiece. Do you know which tissue you can remove with a vitreous cutter and the phacoemulsification handpiece? This is an important knowledge for this case. With the vitreous cutter, you can remove cortex, epinucleus and a soft nucleus. You cannot remove a dense nucleus or a thick capsular fibrosis. With the phacoemulsification handpiece you can remove a dense nucleus and a thick capsular fibrosis. A rock-hard nucleus is difficult to remove by a phacoemulsification handpiece. To remove a rock-hard nucleus, it is advisable to perform a removal with the SICS technique.

Remark   Use always Irrigation and Aspiration from the phaco machine. Do *not* use a separate bottle. A separate bottle results in dangerous IOP fluctuations. The aspiration tubing is attached to the anterior vitreous cutter and the phacoemulsification handpiece and the irrigation tubing is attached to an infusion line which is inserted in a trocar cannula at pars plana.

Chandelier Light   I perform dropped nucleus surgery always with a chandelier light. Why? I want to work with two free hands. I elevate the nucleus with a Charles flute needle, hold it in the middle of the eye and then I cut it with the vitreous cutter. If you choose to work without chandelier light, then you have the light fiber in one hand and the phacoemulsification handpiece in the other hand. The vitreous cutter aspirates the nuclear fragments directly from the retina and doing this you may injure the retina and the choroid. Alternatively, you can elevate the nucleus with a PFCL bubble in order to protect the posterior pole.

The Surgery

Instruments
1. 23G-port trocar system
2. 120D lens
3. Anterior vitreous cutter

Individual Steps
1. 23G, 25G or 27G 3-port system with chandelier light fiber
2. Anterior vitrectomy via pars plana
3. Removal of residual cortex from the lens capsule via paracentesis
4. Vitrectomy, if necessary PVD
5. 20G sclerotomy at 9 o'clock
6. maybe: PFCL for macula protection
7. Emulsification of the nucleus with phacoemulsification handpiece and flute needle
8. Closure of 20G sclerotomy
9. Peripheral vitrectomy
10. Implantation of an intraocular lens
11. Removal of trocar cannulas

The Surgery Step-by-Step: (Figs. 20.14, 20.15, and 20.16)
1. 3-port system with chandelier light fiber

After insertion of 3 trocars we insert a chandelier light fiber, because we work bimanually in step 7 and 9.

2. Anterior vitrectomy via pars plana
3. Removal of residual cortex from the lens capsule via paracentesis
4. Vitrectomy, if necessary PVD

The anterior vitreous is cut with the vitreous cutter via pars plana. Make circular movements with the vitreous cutter. The vitreous cutter port points backwards towards the posterior pole in order to avoid a damage of the lens capsule. Aspirate then the residual cortex with the vitreous cutter via a paracentesis. Alternatively, you can use two I/A hand pieces. It is important that you switch the vitreous cutter to aspiration and not to cutting. Otherwise you risk destroying the anterior capsule. If the lens capsule is free from the cortex, continue with a core vitrectomy from pars plana.

5. 20G sclerotomy at 9 o'clock

Then open the conjunctiva at 9 o'clock in the area of the sclerotomy and perform a non-lamellar (perpendicular) 20G sclerotomy with the V-lance (Fig. 20.14). This sclerotomy is used for the phacoemulsification handpiece and closed as soon as the nucleus is removed, in order to avoid leakage from the sclerotomy.

6. maybe: PFCL for macula protection
7. Emulsification of the nucleus with phacoemulsification handpiece and flute needle

The settings for phacoemulsification are: Low aspiration (approximately 100 mmHg) or sculpting mode. Inject next a small PFCL bubble to protect the macula. Soft lens material can be removed first with the vitreous cutter. For hard lens fragments, you can use the flute needle in your left hand and the phacoemulsification handpiece in the right hand. Aspirate the lens fragments with the flute needle,

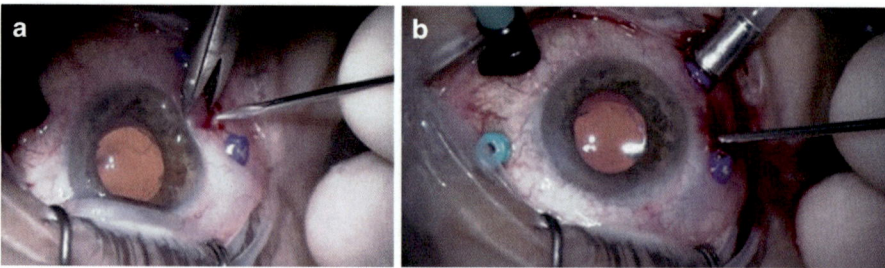

Fig. 20.14 The sclerotomy for the phacoemulsification handpiece is placed at 9 o'clock for right hand dominant surgeons (**a**). Open the conjunctiva and perform a perpendicular sclerotomy (**b**)

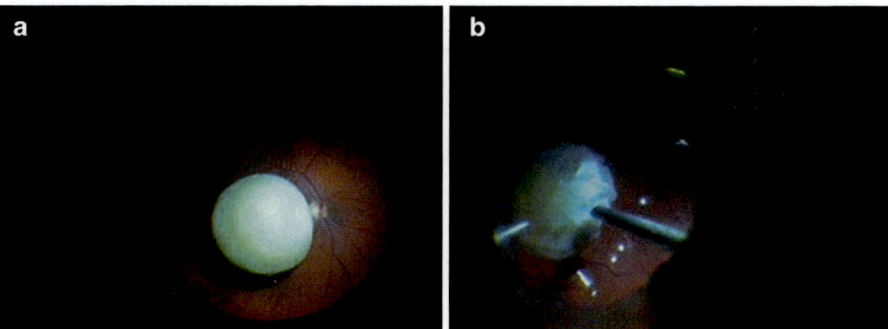

Fig. 20.15 (**a**) A luxated white nucleus secondary to trauma for 20 years ago. (**b**) Emulsification of a nucleus with phacoemulsification handpiece. A PFCL bubble was injected to protect the posterior pole

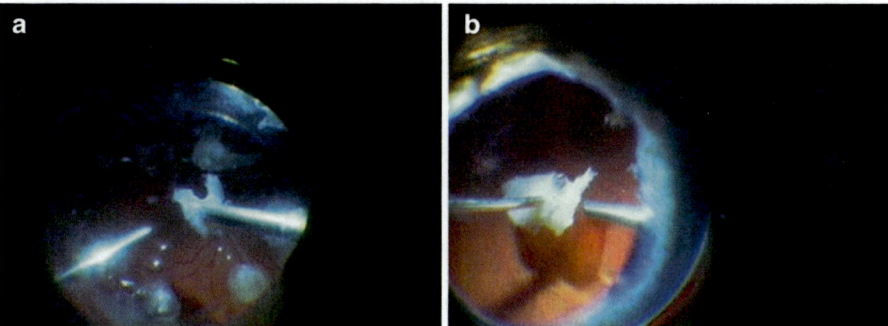

Fig. 20.16 (**a**) Many small nuclear fragments. Every fragment has to be removed. (**b**) The left hand fixates the fragment with a backflush instrument and the right hand removes it with the phacoemulsification handpiece. The phacoemulsification handpiece is a dangerous instrument which can cause severe retinal and choroidal damage

move the needle to the central vitreous cavity and emulsify them there safely with the phacoemulsification handpiece (Figs. 20.15 and 20.16). This procedure is performed repeatedly until all the lens fragments are removed.

If you perform this procedure without flute needle (only with the phacoemulsification handpiece), there is a risk that during the frequent aspiration of the lens fragments with the phacoemulsification handpiece you may injure the retina (retinal break) or the choroid (choroidal hemorrhage). In addition, the frequent aspiration of the lens fragments clogs the vitreous cutter. If the suction is not working properly the risk is increased to induce damage to the retina or choroid. In this case, it is advisable to inject a PFCL bubble in order to protect the posterior pole.

Remark The normal phaco needle may be too short to reach the posterior pole. In this case you need a Charles flute needle or PFCL to elevate the nuclear fragments.

Tips and Tricks

Dropped nucleus: The difficulty of this step is that the nucleus is located on the posterior pole so that a damage of the retina is easily induced. Two advices: (1) Inject a PFCL bubble to (a) protect the macula and (b) elevate the nucleus. (2) Work bimanual so that one hand can fixate the nucleus and the other hand can remove it.

8. Closure of 20G sclerotomy

The 20G sclerotomy must be sutured with a Vicryl 6–0 interrupted stitch or a Vicryl 8–0 cross stitch.

9. Peripheral vitrectomy

The phacoemulsification handpiece breaks the nucleus in many small pieces which are dispersed all over the posterior segment. These fragments must be removed meticulously, because every nucleus fragment which remains may cause a postoperative sterile uveitis. The most lens fragments are located in the vitreous base at 6 o'clock. In order to visualize and remove them you need to indent the vitreous with the scleral depressor. Use for this procedure a chandelier light.

Tips and Tricks

The trimming of the vitreous base is an important step because a *residual nuclear fragment* will cause a postoperative sterile uveitis. Conclusion: Do not be satisfied after removal of the large nucleus but after complete removal of all small fragments.

10. Implantation of the IOL
11. Removal of trocar cannulas

If more than two third of the anterior capsule are intact, the lens can be implanted into the sulcus ("haptic out, optic in"). If not, fixate a 3-piece IOL to the sclera or implant an iris-fixated IOL (Verisyse®).

Tips and Tricks

1-piece IOL vs 3-piece IOL: Do not implant a 1-piece IOL into the sulcus because the haptics cause a focal depigmentation of the iris resulting in a secondary pigment glaucoma. This does not happen with a 3-piece IOL. The reason for this is that a 1-piece haptic has sharp edges and a 3-piece haptic is round.

References

1. Ruiz-Moreno JM, Barile S, Montero JA. Phacoemulsification in the vitreous cavity for retained nuclear lens fragments. Eur J Ophthalmol. 2006;16(1):40–5.
2. Soliman Mahdy M, Eid MZ, Shalaby KA, Hegazy HM. Intravitreal phacoemulsification with pars plana vitrectomy for management of posteriorly dislocated nucleus or lens fragments. Eur J Ophthalmol. 2010;20(1):115–9.
3. Schaal S, Barr CC. Management of retained lens fragments after cataract surgery with and without pars plana vitrectomy. J Cataract Refract Surg. 2009;35(5):863–7. https://doi.org/10.1016/j.jcrs.2008.12.030.

Chapter 21
Posterior Dislocated IOL

A complete luxation of an IOL onto the posterior pole occurs in vitrectomized eyes (Fig. 21.1). It is very unusual in eyes with intact vitreous. The most difficult part of the surgery is the extraction of the IOL from the posterior pole. I will present a simple technique which is easy to learn. After extraction of the IOL a secondary

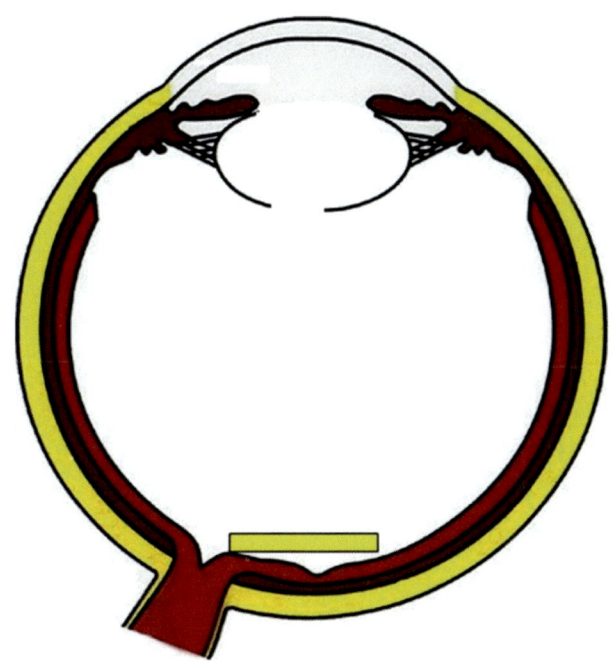

Fig. 21.1 *Posterior dislocated IOL:* The IOL has luxated onto the posterior pole. A vitrectomy is required. Even this surgery is possible with a phacoemulsification machine

---

Electronic Supplementary Material The online version of this chapter (https://doi.org/10.1007/978-3-030-36093-1_21) contains supplementary material, which is available to authorized users.

IOL implantation is performed; scleral fixated with Yamane or Agarwal technique or an Artisan IOL implantation.

The Videos 16.2, 21.1, 21.2, 21.3, and 21.4 demonstrate the surgical management of a posterior dislocated IOL.

21.1 Special Instruments for Extraction of Posterior Dislocated IOL

Endgripping Forceps
Indication: Extraction of IOL from posterior pole into anterior chamber. 23G. DORC 1286.WD06.

Serrated Jaw Forceps (Fig. 21.2)

The Surgery

Instruments
1. Crescent bevel-up knife
2. 15° knife
3. 2.4 mm tunnel knife or Keratome 2.4
4. Caliper
5. IOL implantation forceps (AMO, USA)
6. Enclavation spatula (Geuder, Germany)
7. 20G or 23G Serrated jaw forceps
8. 23G endgripping forceps

Material
Acetylcholine (Miochol)
   Iris claw IOL (Artisan®, Verisyse®)
   Maybe: Triamcinolone

Fig. 21.2 A 23G intravitreal serrated jaws forceps (DORC). Indication: Extraction of the subluxated IOL from the anterior chamber. 20G or 23G. DORC. 1286.C06

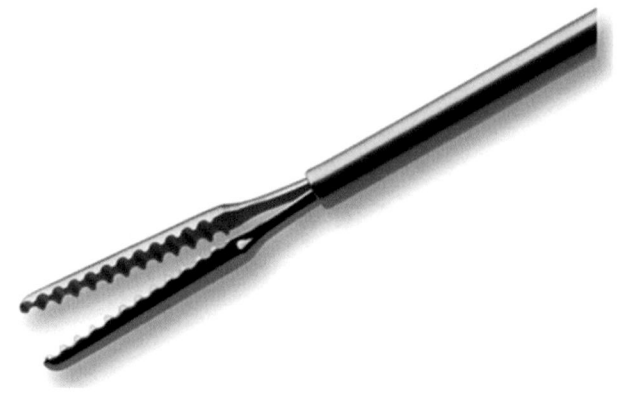

Individual Steps

1. Three 23G trocars
2. Paracentesis at 3 and 9 o'clock
3. Scleral frown incision and a scleral tunnel dissection
4. Extraction of a posterior dislocated IOL
5. Injection of Miochol
6. Implantation of iris fixated IOL (upside down)
7. Closure of the frown incision and conjunctiva

Surgery Step-by-Step: Figs. 21.3, 21.4, 21.5, 21.6, 21.7, and 21.8

1. Three 23G trocars
2. Paracentesis at 3 and 9 o'clock
3. Scleral frown incision and a scleral tunnel dissection

Insert two trocars at the temporal side and one trocar on the nasal side. Continue with a short paracentesis at 3 o'clock and 9 o'clock. The paracentesis is short so that you can reach the peripheral iris with the enclavation spatula.

Fig. 21.3 Mark a 6 mm broad scleral incision with the caliper. The height of the incision is approximately 1.5 mm behind the limbus

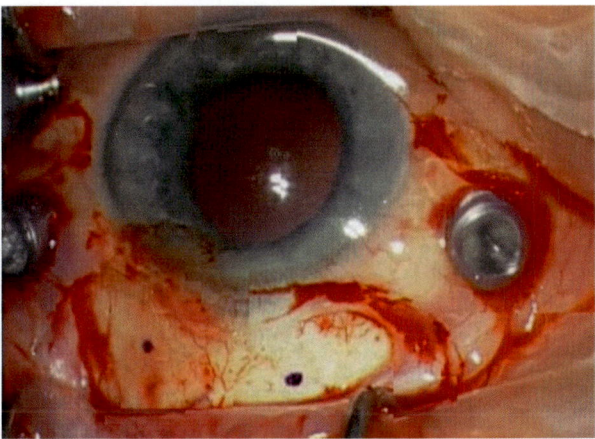

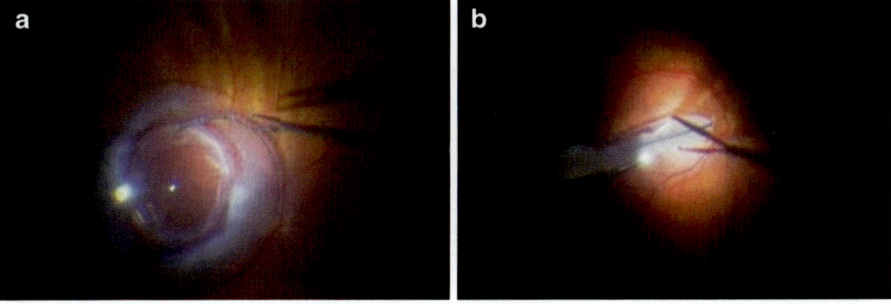

Fig. 21.4 (**a**) Grasp the dislocated IOL and place it upright. (**b**) Fixate the IOL upright with the light pipe and re-grasp the IOL at the haptic or optic edge

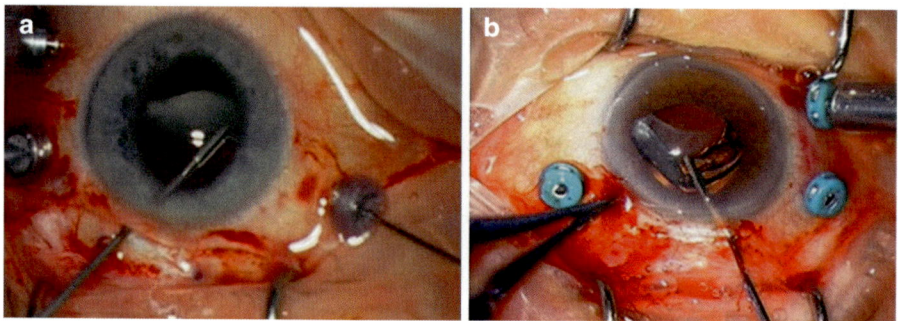

Fig. 21.5 (**a**) Fixate the IOL in the pupil and grasp it with a second (serrated jaws) forceps and release the first forceps. (**b**) Then remove the IOL with the serrated jaws forceps

Fig. 21.6 Extract the IOL together with capsular bag with serrated jaws forceps

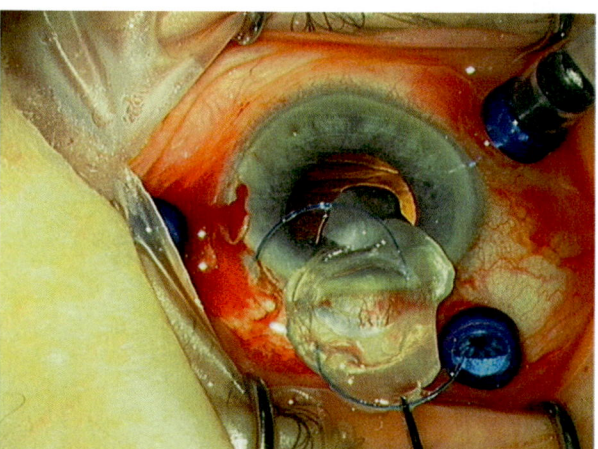

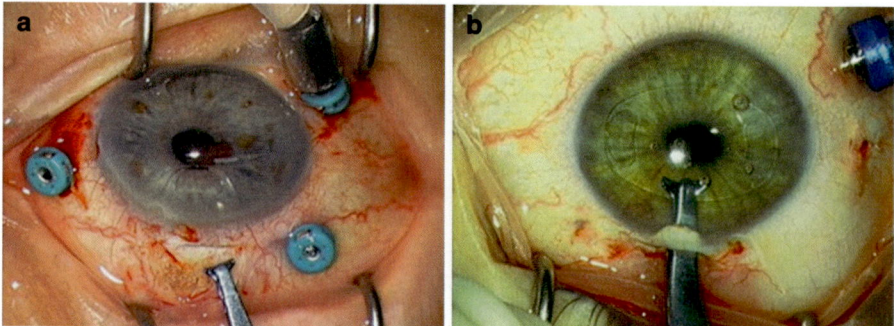

Fig. 21.7 (**a**) Turn the iris-claw IOL upside down for implantation and implant it with the IOL implantation forceps (AMO). (**b**) Centrate the IOL and fixate it with the IOL implantation forceps (AMO)

Fig. 21.8 Note the enclavated iris tissue at 3 and 9 o'clock

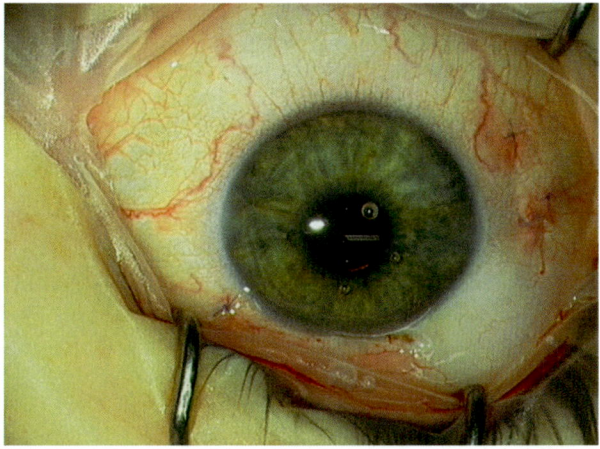

Continue with the frown incision. Perform a limbal peritomy from 11 to 1 o'clock with Westcott scissors and cauterize the bleeding vessels. Then mark a 6-mm wide incision (not wider!) with a caliper (Fig. 21.3). The arc of the incision should be approximately 1–2 mm behind the limbus. Dissect a 50% scleral thickness deep limbus parallel incision with a 15° knife. Then dissect a scleral tunnel with the crescent angled bevel up knife and open finally the anterior chamber with a 2.4 mm blade. Note: Enter the anterior chamber with the 2.4 mm blade in the clear cornea in order to avoid an intracameral bleeding and to create an inner lip valve.

4. Extraction of a posterior dislocated IOL

Instrumentation
Dominant hand: Endgripping forceps
  Non-dominant hand: Light fiber

If the eye is vitrectomized and the IOL is located on the posterior pole, then you have to lift it up (Fig. 21.4). Grasp a part of the lens capsule with the 23G endgripping forceps so that the IOL is standing up (Fig. 21.4a). Support the upright standing IOL with the light pipe and then grasp the IOL again at the edge of the optic or even better at the haptic (Fig. 21.4b). Then lift the IOL up to pupillary plane and flick out the BIOM.

Instrumentation
Dominant hand: Endgripping forceps.
  Non-dominant hand: Serrated jaws forceps.

Then insert the serrated jaws forceps through the main incision and grab the IOL (Fig. 21.5a). Release the first intravitreal forceps and extract the IOL with the serrated jaws forceps (Fig. 21.5b). Alternatively, insert the serrated jaws forceps through a paracentesis and grab the IOL. Withdraw the first intravitreal forceps and reinsert it through the main incision. Grab the IOL with the endgripping forceps, withdraw the serrated jaws forceps (from the paracentesis) and extract the IOL (Fig. 21.6).

Tips and Tricks
Difficult IOL in-the-bag extraction from posterior pole: Inject a small bubble of PFCL to elevate the IOL and to protect the macula. Grab the IOL.

The next step is the secondary IOL implantation. Many techniques are possible. We will show here the implantation of an iris-claw IOL.

5. Injection of Miochol

Inspect then the periphery for retinal tears. The next step is pupil constriction. Before implantation of an iris claw IOL, the pupil must be constricted. Inject first acetylchloline (Miochol®) and then viscoelastics (Viscoat®) into the anterior chamber. Using an IOL forceps (AMO) place the IOL upside down onto the iris (Fig. 21.7a).

6. Implantation of iris fixated IOL (upside down)

Instrumentation
Dominant hand: IOL implantation forceps (Abbott)
   Non-dominant hand: Enclavation spatula

Close the infusion line during IOL implantation. Centrate the IOL with a manipulator (e.g. push-pull) inside the anterior chamber. Grasp the IOL at the edge with the IOL implantation forceps (Abbott) (Fig. 21.7b). Flip the IOL to the right so that the IOL is partially behind the iris and then to flip it to the left so that the IOL is completely behind the iris. Hold the IOL now in the middle of the pupil. Do not move it to the left or right.

Take then the enclavation spatula in your left hand. Lift the IOL a little bit up, so that the iris claws creates an elevated impression behind the iris tissue. Then insert the spatula in the 3 o'clock paracentesis and clamp the iris tissue between the iris-claws. Then the hands for the implantation forceps have to be switched. This maneuver should be thoroughly practiced preoperatively. Then take the enclavation spatula in your right hand and perform the same maneuver at 9 o'clock. Remove finally the implantation forceps and open the infusion line to achieve normotension. A retropupillary implantation requires no iridectomy.

7. Closure of the frown incision and conjunctiva

Suture the frown incision with a Vicryl 8–0 cross stitch and the conjunctiva with a Vicryl 8–0 interrupted stitch (Fig. 21.8).

Postoperative Treatment for Conventional Vitrectomy Atropine x1 for 2 weeks, combined Dexamethasone-Gentamicin drops 5x daily for 2 weeks and 3x daily for third week. After that no drops. In case of aphakia: Atropine drops 1x daily for 2 weeks. In case of Artisan IOL: No mydriatics.

Complications
Complete iris-claw IOL dislocation: The complete dislocation of an iris-claw IOL is very unusual. It may happen postoperatively secondary to a trauma.
   Partial dislocation of an iris-claw IOL (on the nasal side) (Fig. 21.9): The pupil is not dilated with mydriatics. Insert two trocar cannulas at 7 and 9 o'clock. Perform a 2,4 mm corneal incision at 12 o'clock. Insert the vitreous cutter at pars plana,

Fig. 21.9 Elevate the dislocated Artisan IOL from pars plana and place it on top of the iris

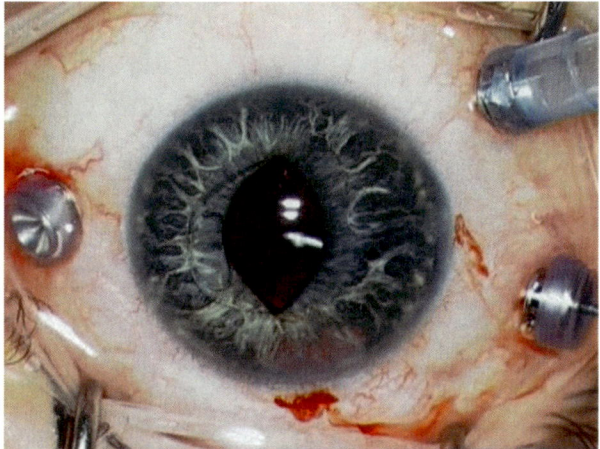

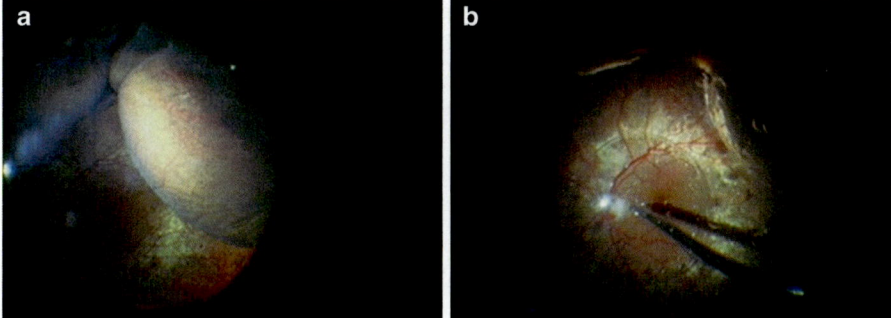

Fig. 21.10 (**a**) A dreaded complication: Choroidal detachment. The reason is the big main incision and pressure fluctuations during manipulations at the main incision. It is therefore important to (1) perform a 6 mm incision (not wider) and (2) close the infusion and fill the anterior chamber with viscoelastics (Viscoat®) when working in the anterior chamber. (**b**) In case of a shallow choroidal detachment an air tamponade is sufficient. In case of a highly bullous choroidal detachment it is advisable to inject PFCL and then perform a PFCL × 1000 csts silicone oil exchange

elevate the IOL and place the loose part on top of the iris. This maneuver is difficult. Remark: Be extremely careful as this maneuver is partly a blind procedure. Then grab the IOL with an IOL forceps from the main incision at 12 o'clock, flip the IOL behind the iris and enclavate the iris tissue (see Video 21.1).

Postoperative inflammation due to traumatic surgery, which occurs only in the learning phase. Do not enclavate too much iris tissue. It may cause ocular pain. In order to avoid this side effect, use the thin enclavation spatula from Sekundo from Geuder.

Choroidal detachment (Fig. 21.10): The cause is the big main incision and pressure fluctuations during manipulations at the main incision. Make the main incision not wider than 6 mm and perform an even cut so that the scleral lips are attached. A shallow choroidal detachment will resorb on its own after 2–3 months. In case of a highly bullous choroidal detachment, inject PFCL and then perform a PFCL × 1000 csts silicone oil exchange.

Chapter 22
Scleral Fixation of a 3-Piece IOL

The Videos 21.3 and 22.1 demonstrate the surgical technique of scleral fixation of an IOL:

Introduction

A fixation of an IOL with sutures is performed seldom nowadays. An intrascleral or iris fixation are more popular nowadays. The scleral fixation with sutures, however, is required for some IOLs such as a pigmented iris IOL (Opthec, NL; Morcher, Germany). This technique is also helpful in case of a partially dislocated IOL. We will demonstrate a technique for the scleral fixation of a partially dislocated IOL as well as for a secondary implanted IOL.

Material

1. Polypropylene 10–0 suture with curved needle (i.e. Alcon. Polypropylene, blue monofilament, double armed. 8,065,307,601 or Ethilon 9091G with LS ultima needle)
2. 3-piece IOL (Alcon MA60AC, ABBOTT Sensar AR40e)

Individual Steps

1. Limbal peritomy at 3 and 9 o'clock

Scleral fixation of intraocular IOL:

2. Two sclerotomies (1.5 mm posterior to the limbus) at 3 and 9 o'clock
3. Extraction of a haptic at 3 o'clock, place a suture onto the haptic and push it back into the eye. The same procedure at 9 o'clock.

Scleral fixation of extraocular IOL:

4. Insert a 10–0 polypropylen suture from 3 to 9 o'clock

Electronic Supplementary Material The online version of this chapter (https://doi.org/10.1007/978-3-030-36093-1_22) contains supplementary material, which is available to authorized users.

U. Spandau, *Trocar Surgery for Cataract Surgeons*,
https://doi.org/10.1007/978-3-030-36093-1_22

5. Extract the suture from main incision and cut in two halves
6. Fasten each half to the haptics of the IOL
7. Insert IOL
8. Suture the haptic suture in a snake shape to the sclera
9. Close the conjunctiva, removal of the trocars

The Surgery Step-by-Step
1. Limbal peritomy at 3 and 9 o'clock

Use a pars plana infusion or an anterior chamber maintainer. Open the conjunctiva at 3 and 9 o'clock to make space for one sclerotomy and a scleral suture, i.e. approximately from 2 to 4 o'clock and from 8 to 10 o'clock. Then cauterize the bleeding vessels.

Scleral fixation of intraocular IOL:

2. Two sclerotomies (1.5 mm posterior to the limbus) at 3 and 9 o'clock
3. Extraction of a haptic at 3 o'clock, place a suture onto the haptic and push it back into the eye. The same procedure at 9 o'clock

In case of a 3-piece IOL fasten the suture in the middle of the haptic and in case of a 1-piece IOL at the end of the haptic.

In the area of the sulcus, 1.5 mm posterior to the limbus, perform an approx. 1.3 mm sclerotomy (Fig. 22.1a). The sclerotomy must be perpendicular (i.e. approximately 90° to the sclera), in order not to injure the iris. Via the sclerotomy at 3 o'clock grasp a haptic with an Eckardt forceps (Fig. 22.1b) and pull it out of the eye. Cut a 10–0 polypropylene suture with two curved needles in two halves. Then fasten a 10–0 prolene suture to the haptic and insert the haptic back into the eye. Perform the same maneuver at the 9 o'clock sclerotomy. After the haptic has been pushed back, center the IOL by pulling carefully on both sutures.

Scleral fixation of extraocular IOL:

4. Insert a 10–0 polypropylen suture from 3 to 9 o'clock.
5. Extract the suture from main incision and cut in two halves.

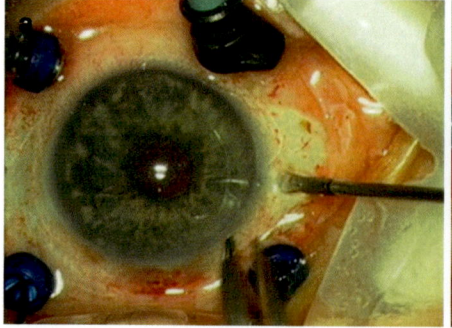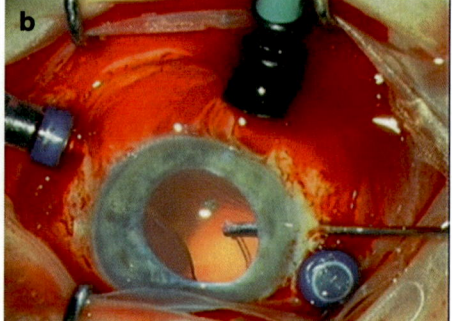

Fig. 22.1 (**a**) A sclerotomy with a V-lance (Alcon) 1.5 mm behind the limbus. (**b**) Grab the end of the haptic and extract it through the sclerotomy

6. Fasten each half to the haptics of the IOL.
7. Insert IOL.

If you want to implant a new IOL the technique is a bit different. Pierce a straight needle transsclerally (Polypropylene 10–0 with straight needle, Alcon) at 3 or 9 o'clock and 1,5 mm behind the limbus (Fig. 22.2a). Engage from the opposite sclera a 27G cannula which is fastened to a syringe. Catch the straight needle with the 27G cannula and pull it out. Now you have a 10–0 polypropylen suture from 3 to 9 o'clock. Grab the suture from the main incision with intravitreal forceps (Fig. 22.2b), pull the suture outside the eye and cut it in two halves. Fasten each end to one haptic of IOL. Then implant the IOL with an IOL forceps (Fig. 22.2c). You cannot use an injector. Centrate the IOL by pulling on both sutures. Then fasten the sutures with a snake suture to the sclera as follows:

8. Suture the haptic suture in a snake shape to the sclera.

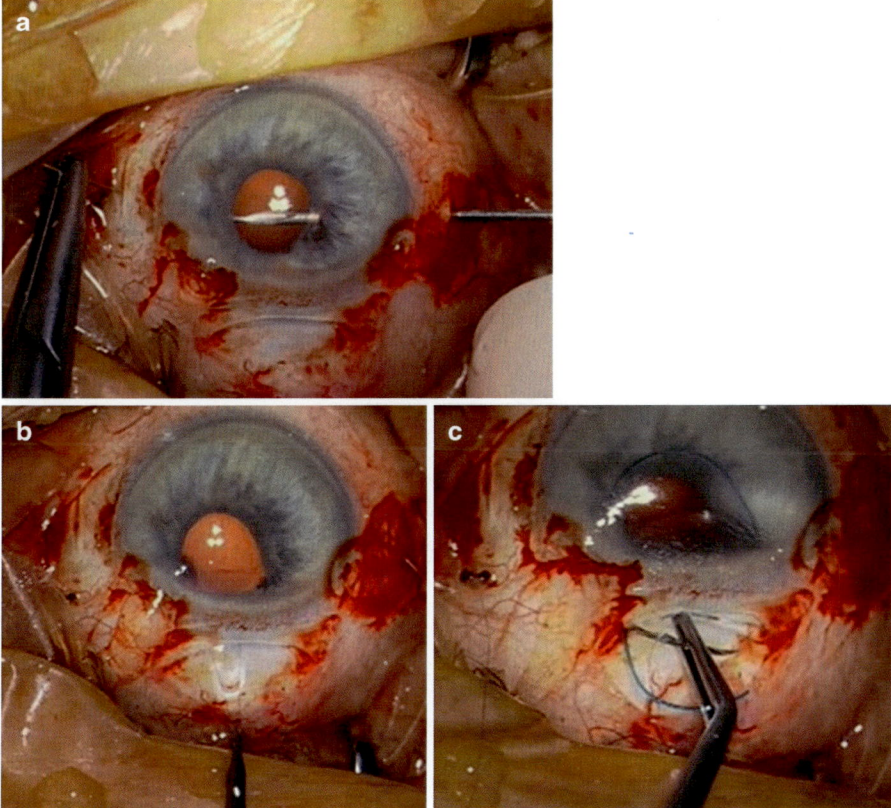

Fig. 22.2 (**a**) Insert a 10–0 polypropylen suture from 3 to 9 o'clock. (**b**) Extract the middle of the suture from the main incision and cut it in two halves. (**c**) Fasten both ends to the haptics and implant the IOL

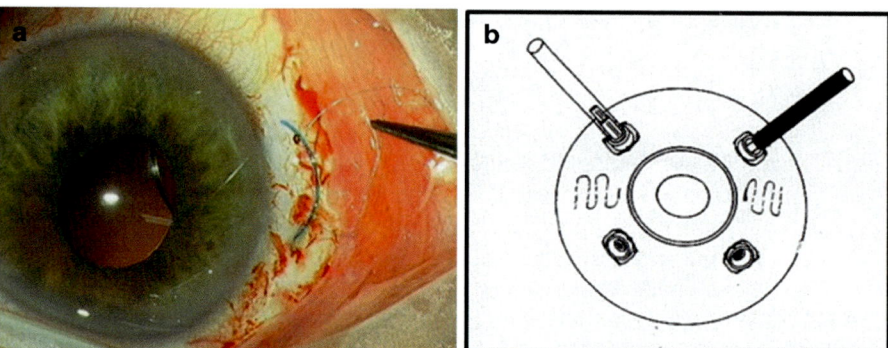

Fig. 22.3 (**a**) Tie one end of a 10–0 prolene 10.0 suture to one haptic. This suture has one straight needle. Then same maneuver on the other side. (**b**) 5x snake shaped stitch. A knot is not necessary

Different techniques are now possible. Move the needle in a shape snake 5 times through the sclera and then cut off the suture without a knot. A knot can cause a disturbing foreign body sensation to the patient (Fig. 22.3). Alternatively, you can prepare a scleral flap, fasten the suture to the sclera and place the knot under the scleral flap.

9. Close the conjunctiva, removal of the trocars.

The conjunctiva is closed with an 8–0 Vicryl stitch. The sclerotomies do not need to be sutured.

Part V
General Surgical Techniques

Chapter 23
Small Incision Cataract Surgery
(SICS = Modified ECCE)

The Video 23.1 demonstrates the surgical technique of a SICS surgery (modified ECCE).

If the nucleus is too dense for phacoemulsification and you risk a corneal decompensation, you can remove the nucleus faster and with fewer complications in toto. An excellent technique is SICS (modified ECCE). The main difference between SICS and ECCE is the main incision (Fig. 23.1). In ECCE a limbal incision from 10 o'clock to 2 o'clock is performed; in SICS a frown incision of the sclera is performed. A frown incision is tighter and more stable than a corneal incision. A suture is usually not necessary. We prefer to suture the frown incision with a Vicryl 8–0 cross stitch. We recommend performing the surgery in peribulbar anaesthesia.

Fig. 23.1 SICS surgery.
8 mm wide frown incision

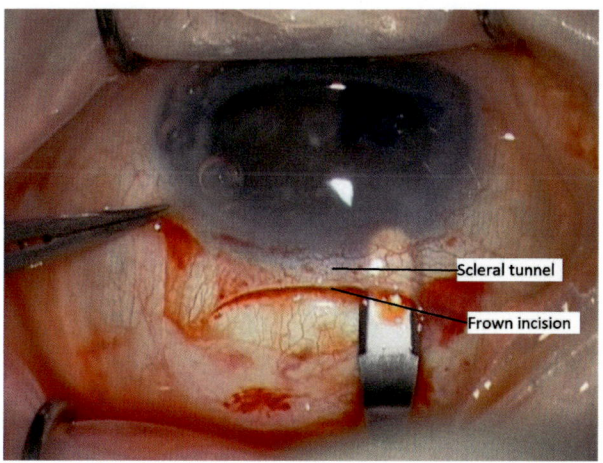

Scleral tunnel

Frown incision

Electronic Supplementary Material The online version of this chapter (https://doi.org/10.1007/978-3-030-36093-1_23) contains supplementary material, which is available to authorized users.

23.1   Standard Instruments for SICS

Phaco Set
Phaco handpiece and IOL injector are not needed.

Frown Incision
Westcott scissors (Fig. 23.2).

Caliper
Indication: Marking of main incision and sclerotomy. The main incision for the implantation of an iris-fixated PMMA IOL is 6 mm wide. Caliper by Castroviejo, Geuder 19,135.
    Crescent angled bevel up knife (Fig. 23.3).

Rotation of Nucleus
Y-manipulator or nucleus rotator (Fig. 23.4).

Fig. 23.2 Westcott scissors. Indication: Limbal peritomy. Geuder 19,750

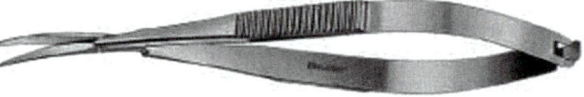

Fig. 23.3 Crescent angled bevel up knife. Indication: Dissection of a scleral tunnel. (Alcon 8,065,990,002, Beaver Visitec 373,835, DORC 51.1118 or Aurosleek crescent bevel up (Aurolab))

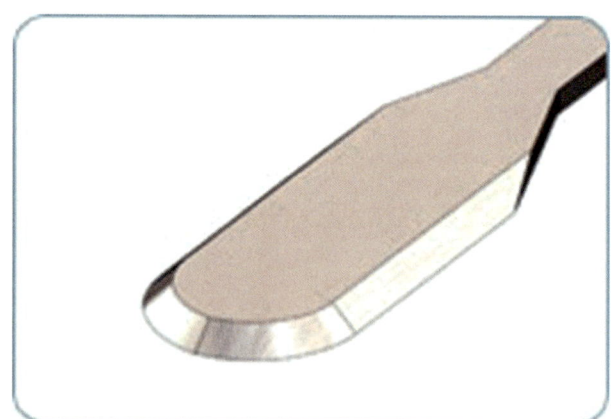

Fig. 23.4 Y-manipulator or nucleus rotator. Indication: Rotation of nucleus, very useful during SICS surgery for luxation of the nucleus into the anterior chamber. Nucleus rotator after Neuhann, Geuder 32,160

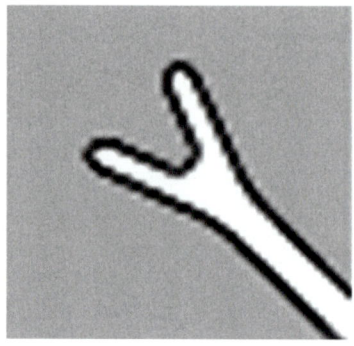

Fig. 23.5 Lens extraction hook. Indication: Extraction of nucleus. Lens extraction hook after Henning/Friedrich, Geuder 32,034

Extraction of Nucleus
Lens extraction hook (Fig. 23.5)

Alternative (1) 27G grey cannula. Bend a 27G cannula to a fish hook. (2) Lens loop or Vectis (Serrated lens loop, Geuder 15,620).

23.2 SICS Surgery

Instruments
1. I/A
2. Lens nucleus rotator
3. 15° knife
4. Crescent bevel up knife
5. 2.4 mm tunnel knife also known as keratome
6. Caliper
7. Lens extraction hook (Geuder, Germany) or serrated lens loop (Geuder, Germany)

Individual Steps
1. Capsulorhexis
2. Limbal peritomy
3. Frown incision and scleral tunnel construction
4. Luxation of nucleus into anterior chamber
5. Inflate lens capsule with viscoelastics
6. Rotation of the nucleus into the anterior chamber
7. Extraction of the nucleus
8. I/A
9. Implantation of a 3-piece IOL
10. Suturing of frown incision and conjunctiva

The Surgery Step-by-Step
1. Capsulorhexis

Begin with a paracentesis at 10 and 2 o'clock and inject viscoelastics (Viscoat®) into the anterior chamber. Perform then a large rhexis because the nucleus must be dislocated from the capsular bag (Fig. 23.6).

2. Limbal peritomy
3. Frown incision and scleral tunnel construction

Continue with a limbal peritomy from 11 o'clock to 1 o'clock with a Westcott scissors. Cauterize bleeding vessels and mark an 8 mm wide incision with a caliper (Fig. 23.7a). Perform an arc-shaped and 50% scleral thickness incision with the 15°

Fig. 23.6 Perform a large rhexis. A large rhexis is necessary to luxate the nucleus out of the lens capsule

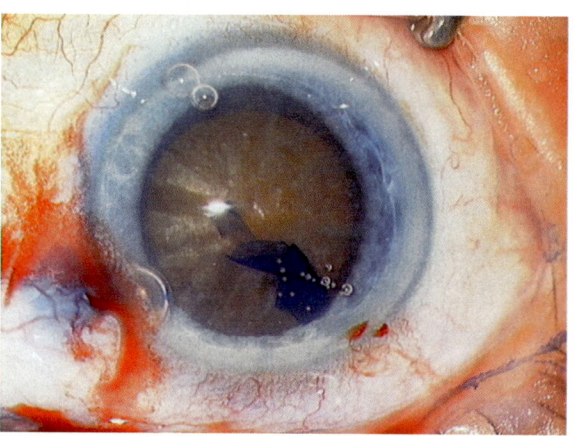

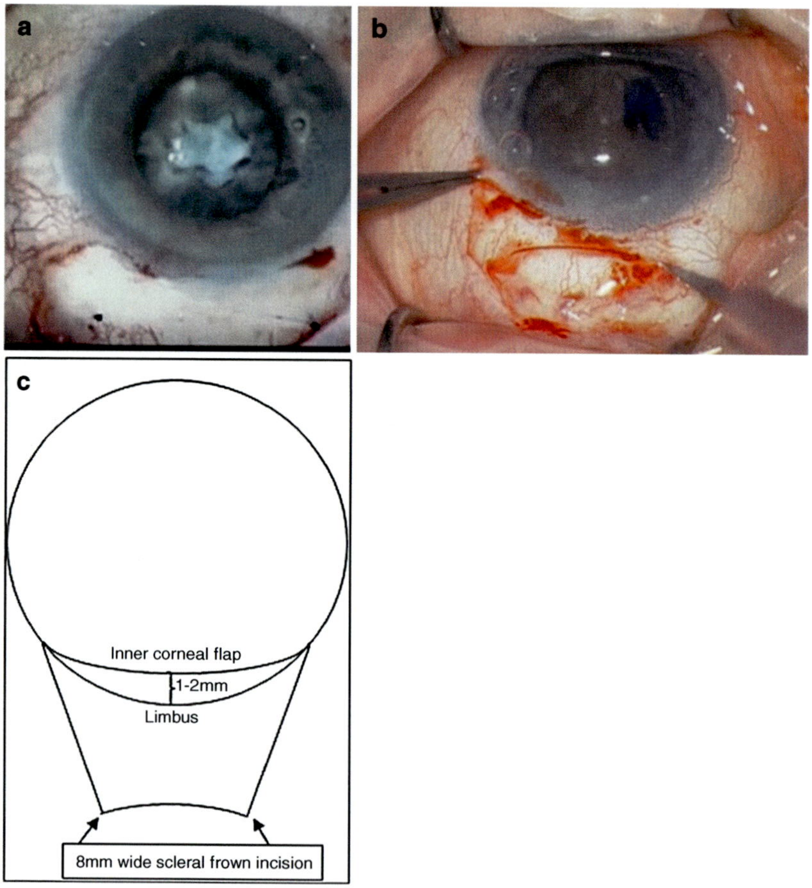

Fig. 23.7 (**a**) Mark an 8 mm long incision on the sclera. (**b**) Perform an 50% scleral thickness incision with the 15° knife. (**c**) Drawing of a frown incision. The incision is 8 mm broad and the tunnel has a "V" shape

knife (Fig. 23.7b). Dissect a scleral tunnel with the crescent angled bevel up knife (Fig. 23.8). Do not dissect too deep (iris prolapse) but not too thin either (flap defect). If the blade is shining through the sclera, it is at the correct depth. Then open the main incision with the 2.4 mm tunnel knife (Fig. 23.8). Move the knife 1–2 mm inside the clear cornea before entering the anterior chamber (Fig. 23.7c). Be aware that the scleral tunnel has a V-shape and not a U-shape like the normal tunnel incision (Fig. 23.7c), i.e. the scleral tunnel widens from the sclera to the anterior chamber.

Tips and Tricks
Caution: The scleral tunnel in SICS surgery has a "V" shape. The scleral tunnel in iris-claw implantation surgery has the shape of a "U" (Fig. 23.7c).

4. Luxation of nucleus into anterior chamber
5. Inflate lens capsule with viscoelastics
6. Rotation of the nucleus into the anterior chamber

   Non-dominant hand: Y-manipulator
   Dominant hand: Viscoelastics syringe
   Continue with hydrodissection. If the rhexis is large enough, the nucleus prolapses out due to hydrodissection from the capsular bag. If the nucleus fails to prolapse from the capsular bag during hydrodissection then you need to luxate the nucleus manually into the anterior chamber. Place the tip of the Y-manipulator at the superior edge of the nucleus and lift the nucleus up. Inject with the other hand viscoelastics (Viscoat®) behind the nucleus in order to inflate the lens capsule (Fig. 23.9). Then lift the nucleus completely into the anterior chamber. It is important to inject viscoelastics behind the nucleus in order to avoid a posterior capsular defect.

7. Extraction of the nucleus

   For nucleus extraction use a lens extraction hook (Geuder, Germany). Use alternatively a lens loop. Before extracting the nucleus assure yourself that there

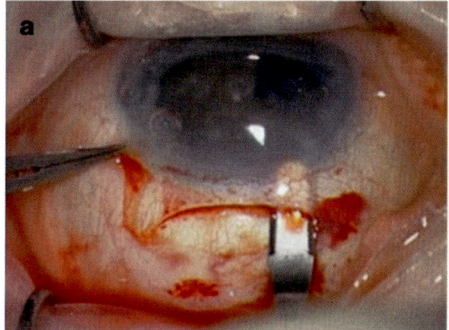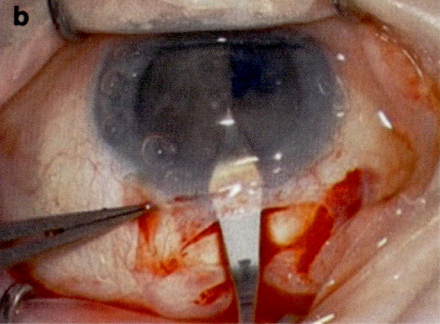

Fig. 23.8 (**a**) Dissect a scleral flap with a crescent bevel up knife. If the blade of the knife is visible through the tissue you are on the right level. (**b**) Open the anterior chamber with a 2.4 mm blade. Do not enter the anterior chamber too close to the limbus; otherwise the iris will prolapse

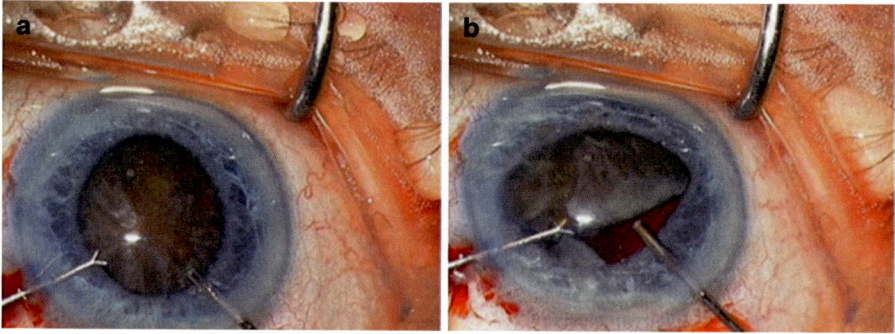

Fig. 23.9 (**a**) The left hand holds a Y-manipulator or Sinskey hook manipulator and the right hand viscoelastics. Place the Y-manipulator on the superior edge of the nucleus. (**b**) Then lift the nucleus up with the Y-manipulator and inject viscoelastics into the open space between nucleus and lens capsule in order to inflate the lens capsule

is viscoelastics (Viscoat®) above and behind the nucleus in order to protect the lens capsule and the endothelium. Then insert the fish hook with the hook pointed to the side. Place the hook behind the middle of the nucleus, turn the hook into an upright position and draw the nucleus slowly out (Fig. 23.10). Check first that you did not catch the inferior iris with the fish hook. If the nucleus gets stuck in the frown incision, then do not insist; reinject viscoelastics and enlarge the frown incision with the 2.4 mm tunnel knife and repeat the extraction manoeuvre.

8. I/A
9. Implantation of a 3-piece IOL
10. Suturing of the frown incision and conjunctiva

Continue with I/A. Then implant a 3-piece IOL because of the large rhexis (Fig. 23.11). The IOL requires no folding, because the main incision is sufficient large. Proceed to suture the main incision with a Vicryl 8–0 cross-stitch. If necessary, suture also the conjunctiva (Fig. 23.11). Remove the viscoelastics with I/A from the anterior chamber.

Caution Keep an eye on the frown incision during surgery. Avoid that the incision is gaping because this may lead to a choroidal detachment. Close therefore the incision as soon as possible with a suture.

Summary
Train yourself with the three techniques, phacoemulsification, SICS (modified ECCE) and the saving of a dropping nucleus from pars plana, and you do not need help from a posterior segment surgeon. You are now a cataract surgeon master.

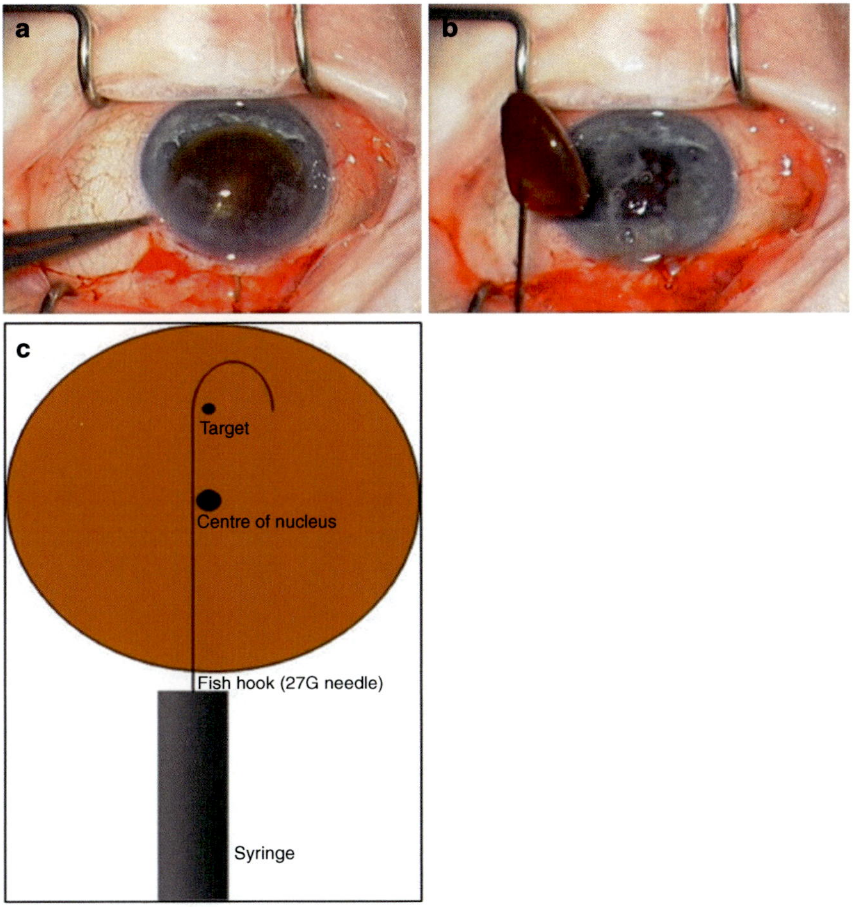

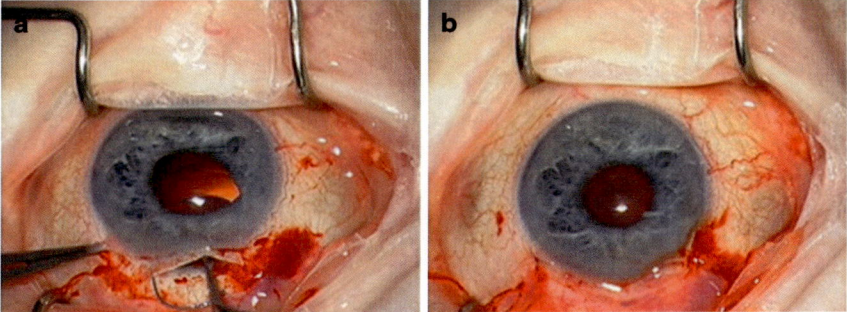

Fig. 23.10 (**a**) Inject viscoelastics between the nucleus and the lens capsule and between the nucleus and the endothelium. Insert the fish hook with the hook facing to the right. If you reach the extraction position (see Fig. 23.10c) then turn the cannula so that the hook faces the nucleus. (**b**) Remove the nucleus. (**c**) Drawing: Position the fish hook behind the nucleus as depicted

Fig. 23.11 (**a**) Implant a 3-piece IOL. An injector is not necessary. (**b**) Close the conjunctiva with a Vicryl 8–0 interrupted stitch

Chapter 24
Pars Plana Vitrectomy Step-by-Step

The following chapter describes step-by-step a vitrectomy. The most steps can be performed with a phacoemulsification machine. Separate devices are, however, required such as a light source or a laser photocoagulation device.

The Video 18.1 demonstrates the surgical management of a pars plana vitrectomy.

24.1   Topography in Vitrectomy

The correct topography of the eye during surgery is more difficult than you might expect (Fig. 24.1). The lens is located in front or anterior. The retina is located in the back or posterior. A peripheral break is equivalent to an anterior break and a central break equivalent to a posterior break. You make a sclerotomy <u>not</u> below the limbus, but behind or posterior to the limbus. You move the vitreous cutter from the back (retina) to the front (lens). Hold the Charles flute needle behind the lens (in the front of the eye).

24.2   Intraocular Pressure: Clinical Asessment and Surgical Action

The tonus of the globe is an essential element of anterior and especially of posterior segment surgery. As a surgeon you must be able to assess the tonus of the globe and take adequate actions.

Electronic Supplementary Material The online version of this chapter (https://doi.org/10.1007/978-3-030-36093-1_24) contains supplementary material, which is available to authorized users.

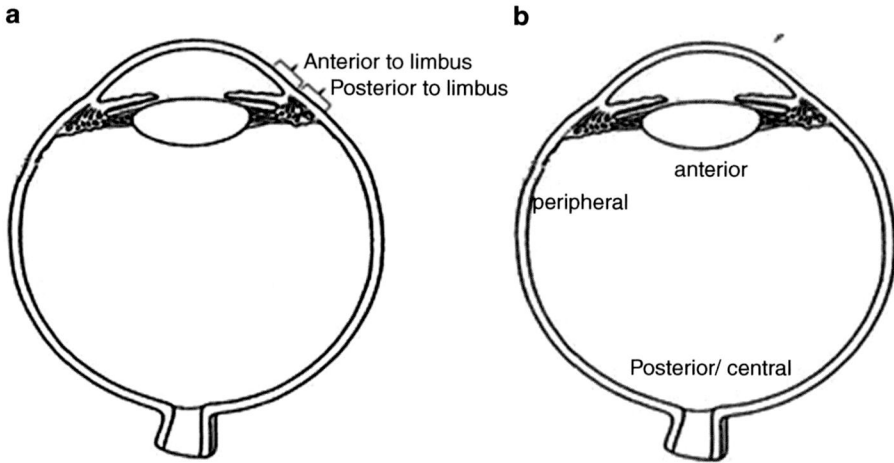

Fig. 24.1 (**a**) A trocar is inserted *posterior* (*or behind*) to the limbus. (**b**) The lens is located *anterior* and the macula is located *posterior*. The optic disc is located posterior in the center of the retina. The vitreous base is located peripherally

Assessment The intraocular pressure can be assessed in the easiest way with the index finger. During posterior segment surgery you check the globe pressure regularly with your index finger. There are also clinical signs for high and low IOP. If the IOP is too high, then the cornea becomes edematous because the endothelium cannot pump out the excess intracorneal fluid. Further signs are an iris prolapses through the corneal incision and a flat anterior chamber. In the posterior segment a high IOP can only be visualized with a non-pulsatile optic disc. A low IOP presents with a globe losing its shape, scleral folds occur. In addition, a choroidal detachment develops. In the anterior segment there are hardly signs for a low IOP except for folds in the cornea or a gaping scleral tunnel.

Another important factor is the presence of aphakia or not. If aphakia is present, then intraocular fluid can flow freely from posterior to anterior segment and vice versa. *Remark*: A PCR is more or less comparable to aphakia.

In contrast, if a natural lens or in-the-bag IOL is present, then aqueous flows only slowly from posterior to anterior segment and vice versa. For example: In case of aphakia or PCR an anterior chamber maintainer has the same effect as a pars plana trocar infusion because no barrier between anterior and posterior segment is present. If, however, a natural lens or an in-the-bag IOL is present, then an anterior chamber maintainer cannot maintain the IOP in the posterior segment. If you perform in this situation a vitrectomy then an underpressure in the posterior segment will develop. This underpressure may result in a subchoroidal hemorrhage.

Surgical Procedure What to do if the IOP is too high? The simplest surgical procedure is a paracentesis. If a paracentesis is not possible because of a flat anterior chamber, then you can relieve pressure from the posterior segment (via pars plana). This can be achieved with a needle cannula or a vitreous cutter. If the IOP is too low, you can increase the IOP by injecting fluid into the anterior chamber or into the posterior chamber (like an intravitreal injection). Assess the effect of your action with the index finger.

24.3 Pars Plana Vitrectomy Step-by-Step

In the following section, a standard pars plana vitrectomy is explained. As in a cookbook the ingredients (instruments, dyes, and tamponade) are listed first and then the practical approach is explained in detail step by step. For beginners we recommend only to operate pseudophakic eyes and *not* phakic eyes. The risk to injure the lens in phakic eyes is too high for inexperienced surgeons. See Video 18.1.

Instruments
1. 3-port trocar system
2. Viewing system
3. Light pipe with external light source
4. Anterior vitreous cutter (23G)
5. Scleral depressor
6. Backflush instrument

Dye
Triamcinolone

Tamponade
Air, gas, silicone oil

Individual Steps
1. Insertion of trocar cannulas
2. Phacoemulsification
3. Anterior vitrectomy
4. Focusing of viewing system
5. Core vitrectomy.
6. Induction of posterior vitreous detachment
7. Removal of peripheral vitreous
8. Internal search for retinal breaks
9. Laserphotocoagulation of peripheral breaks
10. Cryotherapy of peripheral breaks
11. Intraoperative tamponade (short term tamponade).
12. Postoperative tamponade (long term tamponade)
13. Removal of trocar cannulas
14. Sclerotomy sutures

The Surgery Step-by-Step
1. Insertion of Trocars

The sclerotomies must be placed in the pars plana (there is no retina). The distance of the sclerotomies to the limbus is 3.5 mm in pseudophakic eyes and aphakics

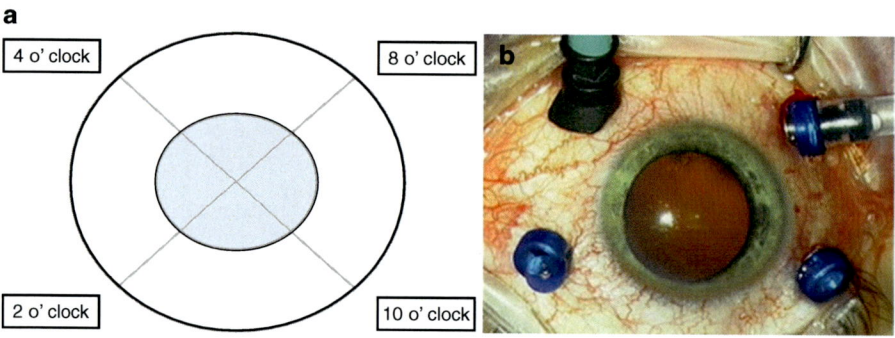

Fig 24.2 (**a**) Drawing of a 4-port vitrectomy in a right eye: Two instrument ports, one infusion port and one chandelier light. (**b**) Photo of a 4-port vitrectomy: Instrument ports, infusion port and chandelier light (25G Awh, Synergetics)

and 4.0 mm in phakic eyes. By using a scleral marker, you can measure and mark the sclerotomy. It is recommended that you always (even after the beginner phase) use this scleral marker to avoid unnecessary complications due to misplaced sclerotomies.

The insertion of the trocars is an important step. It may look frightening at the beginning, but it is actually easier than it looks. The infusion trocar is always located inferotemporal: For the left eye at 4 o'clock and for the right eye at 8 o'clock. The other two trocars are located at 2 and 10 o'clock. These two trocars are used for instruments. In some cases, a chandelier light is required. Many surgeons place the chandelier light at the 12 o'clock position. But the chandelier light easily dislocates at this position. We prefer to place the chandelier light at the inferotemporal position (Fig. 24.2). It dislocates very seldom in this position.

Practical procedure (Figs. 24.3 and 24.4) Start always with the infusion port inferotemporally. Take a cotton swab in one hand, a 3.5 mm scleral marker (pseudophakic eye) in the other hand and place the cotton swab posterior (behind) the limbus on the conjunctiva. Pull the conjunctiva a little to the side parallel to the limbus, mark the sclerotomy with the scleral marker. Usually a minor bleeding highlights the sclerotomy site. Take next the trocar handpiece and perform a transconjunctival sclerotomy. The first half of the insertion is 15 degrees parallel to the limbus and the second half upright towards the middle of the eye (perpendicular). Finally, fixate the trocar cannula with the trocar forceps and remove the trocar handpiece.

Hold the infusion cannula with the trocar forceps (DORC, see materials) and insert the closed infusion line. Then ascertain whether the infusion cannula is located in the vitreous cavity: You turn the cannula with the trocar forceps in direction of the cornea until you can recognize with certainty the cannula's location in the vitreous cavity. Alternatively insert the light pipe through the infusion trocar. Then the other trocar cannulas are inserted 2 o'clock and at 10 o'clock with the same procedure.

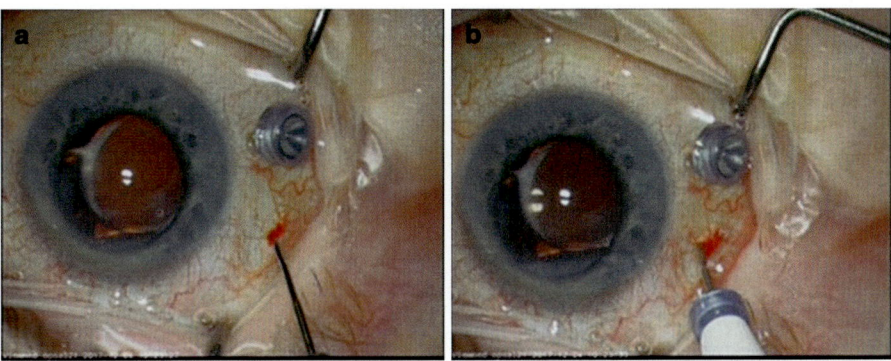

Fig 24.3 (**a**) A small bleeding highlights the sclerotomy site. Insert the trocar at an angle of about 15 degrees parallel to the limbus. (**b**) Insert the first half of the trocar cannula

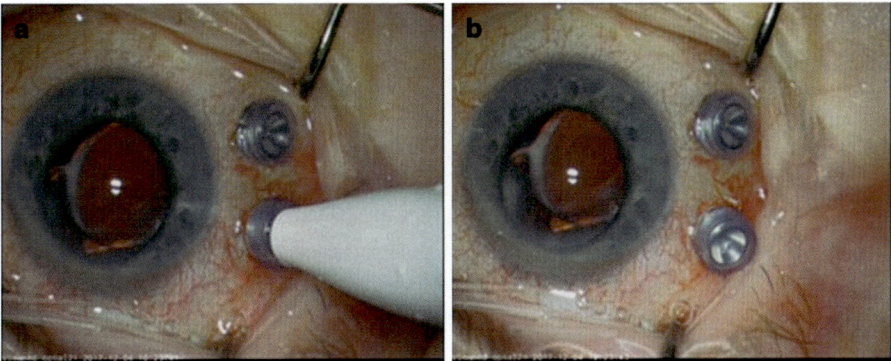

Fig 24.4 (**a**) Insert the second half perpendicular towards the middle of the eye. (**b**) Finally, fixate the trocar cannula with the trocar forceps and remove the trocar handpiece

The procedure concerning the location of the infusion cannula in the vitreous cavity is very important as incorrect positioning of the infusion cannula can cause a number of complications; e.g. subchoroidal positioning can cause a choroidal detachment; subepithelial positioning can cause a detached pars plana and a subretinal positioning can lead to a detached retina (Table 24.1). *Remark:* The infusion line enters the eye first and exits last.

Tips and Tricks
Conjunctival chemosis: If the conjunctiva has been ballooned through the local anesthetic or during previous phacoemulsification then compress the conjunctiva at the sclerotomy site with a trocar forceps or anatomic forceps.

Tips and Tricks
In patients with *narrow lid margins* (for example, children or Asian patients), ports that are placed too superiorly may "disappear" under the upper eyelid. Constantly

Table 24.1 Anatomy of the pars plana (from outside to inside)

Sclera
Pars plana epithelium
Vitreous

moving the eye inferiorly to expose the hidden ports and introduce your instruments can be extremely annoying during the surgery. Place the trocar cannulas more horizontally.

Tips and Tricks

Infusion Cannula

(1) Examination of the inner opening of the infusion cannula before starting the infusion is a must in each and every vitrectomy. Make sure that it is not blocked by ciliary epithelium or intraocular membranes. Opening the infusion whilst the opening is under the ciliary epithelium can within seconds turn a straightforward vitrectomy into a nightmare case.

(2) When you can see that the opening is in the correct position but is blocked by blood or membranes, try to clear the opening from the opposite side with a vitreous cutter. Be careful not to touch the lens during this maneuver in phakic patients. In the case of doubt, remove the infusion port and try a different site for your infusion.

(3) If you are still unsure whether your infusion port is in the right place, introduce the light pipe through the port. You should be able to confirm the correct position even through hemorrhages in the vitreous base.

(4) In very complicated cases when you cannot examine the infusion port (trauma, endophthalmitis), start the vitrectomy with infusion connected to an anterior chamber maintainer. Clear the vitreous immediately behind the lens with a vitreous cutter introduced through the pars plana to clear the view. Then insert the infusion trocar via the pars plana as soon as you can see the vitreous base. Even in such complicated cases, do not open the infusion without confirming that the infusion cannula is in the correct position.

2. Phacoemulsification

We recommend inserting the trocars before phacoemulsification because the globe is very soft after phacoemulsification which makes the insertion of trocars difficult. During phacoemulsification, the infusion is closed.

The phacoemulsification is performed as usual. Regarding the size of your rhexis, it is important to ensure that the edge of the rhexis circularly covers the intraocular lens, as the IOL optic can easily dislocate during vitrectomy in front of the anterior capsule. Therefore, perform a smaller capsulorhexis (4–5 mm). Furthermore, is it advisable to polish the anterior capsule (anterior capsule polishing) to enable a clear view into the periphery. The IOL is usually inserted at the end of the phaco and before the vitrectomy. In difficult cases, some surgeons prefer to insert the IOL at the end of the PPV, because the IOL edge disturbs the view into the periphery. After IOL implantation and irrigation and aspiration hydrate the paracentesis and the tunnel well to ensure a stable anterior chamber during the vitrectomy. If the anterior chamber during vitrectomy is unstable, place a 10–0 nylon X-stitch at the tunnel. This is particularly advisable if significant indentation is planned during the vitrectomy (for example, retinal detachment cases), as indentation may open the corneoscleral wound and displace the IOL.

Important In pseudophakic eyes BSS is used as irrigation fluid and in phakic eyes BSS Plus®. BSS Plus® also contains glutathione, glucose and sodium bicarbonate (see materials list).

Tips and Tricks
Close the *infusion* during an *anterior segment* procedure.

Tips and Tricks
Perform a combined *phaco and vitrectomy* only if you previously have gained considerable experience in performing phacos. This step of the surgery must be performed flawlessly. If you struggle with the phaco, the cornea is likely to opacify during surgery, making retinal manipulations later on extremely challenging. If you damage the bag or the zonules, you run the risk of tamponade prolapse into the anterior chamber.

Tips and Tricks
If you are really running into trouble during the phaco with corneal edema or damage to the lens in cases of elective surgery (macular hole, membrane peeling), think about delaying the vitrectomy part of the procedure until the situation has improved a couple of days later.

Tips and Tricks
Posterior capsular opacification: Should be removed if it reduces visibility. In addition, a YAG-laser capsulotomy is significantly more difficult in vitrectomized eyes. A PCO can be removed from pars plana with the vitreous cutter. Settings: approx. 500 cpm and normal vacuum. Cut a circular hole in the posterior capsule. The IOL cannot be injured by this procedure. A small central capsulotomy is sufficient. A larger capsulotomy is associated with the dangers of IOL dislocation and tamponade prolapse into the anterior chamber.

Tips and Tricks
Frosting/thawing of the IOL may occur during fluid against air exchange (FAX) if the posterior lens capsule is removed within the central area. Apply a thin layer of viscoelastics (Viscoat®) on the posterior surface of the IOL and visualization will improve.

Tips and Tricks
Blood in the anterior chamber: If you experience a bleeding during the PPV into the anterior chamber, you can either aspirate the blood with irrigation or aspiration instruments or inject a viscoelastics (Viscoat®) into the anterior chamber to push the blood to the edge of the anterior chamber and tamponade the bleeding. Ask the scrub nurse to remind you to remove the viscoelastic at the end of the vitrectomy. The removal has to be done before you instill the tamponade.

Tips and Tricks

Blood clots in the anterior chamber: If the bleeding has stopped, extract fibrous strands of blood with intravitreal forceps through a paracentesis.

Tips and Tricks

Hypotony of the globe. If the globe is hypotonous under phacoemulsification or any other situation, then inject BSS to normalize the IOP. Attach a flute needle (from backflush instrument) onto a syringe with BSS. Inject BSS via a trocar cannula into the posterior vitreous cavity in order to normalize the intraocular pressure.

Tips and Tricks

Hypertony of the globe. If the globe is hypertonous under phacoemulsification, then perform a dry vitrectomy. A dry vitrectomy is performed with a closed infusion. Place the vitreous cutter behind the lens and cut. Control constantly the pressure of the globe with your index finger. If the pressure of the globe has become normal, retract the vitreous cutter and continue with phacoemulsification.

3. Anterior vitrectomy

Remove the anterior vitreous of posterior segment. Hold the vitreous cutter behind the posterior capsule and move the cutter in circular fashion while the opening of the cutter is directed downwards in order not to injure the capsule.

As beginner, it is amazing to learn how much vitreous is present in the eye. This can be noticed intraoperatively when air bubbles are trapped in the vitreous behind the lens capsule. These air bubbles cannot be removed with the flute needle but only by removing the vitreous behind the lens capsule. An anterior vitrectomy is easy in pseudophakic patients, in phakic patients it is dangerous because the location of the posterior capsule is difficult to determine. Injury to the posterior capsule is a common beginner's mistake. Therefore, start vitrectomies only in pseudophakic patients.

Tips and Tricks

Vitrectomy in phakic eyes. A paracentesis may be done to make the anterior chamber shallow since the crystalline lens moves anteriorly. Now a removal of the anterior vitreous is easier and safer.

4. Focusing with viewing system

The surgeon or the scrub nurse flicks in the BIOM (Fig. 24.5). Next, the light pipe is introduced in the nasal trocar towards the macula, until the pupil is bright. Then, the inverter is activated, the microscope light turned off and the image is focused.

If you are using the BIOM (Oculus) system, it may be frustrating to adjust the focus at the beginning of vitrectomy. However, if you keep a few rules in mind you will find focusing easy. There are three adjustable parameters: 1. Focus wheel at the BIOM; 2. Focus on foot pedal of the microscope and 3. Zoom on foot pedal of the microscope. (Fig. 24.5). When focusing the image, you should only change the two parameters focus wheel BIOM and focus foot pedal and NOT the zoom. You should only change the zoom when you have a sharp image.

Fig 24.5 A surgical microscope with attached BIOM. Integrated is an inverter, which may be operated manually or by foot pedal. At the front of the BIOM the interchangeable front lenses are attached. The adjustment body can be adjusted with the focus wheel

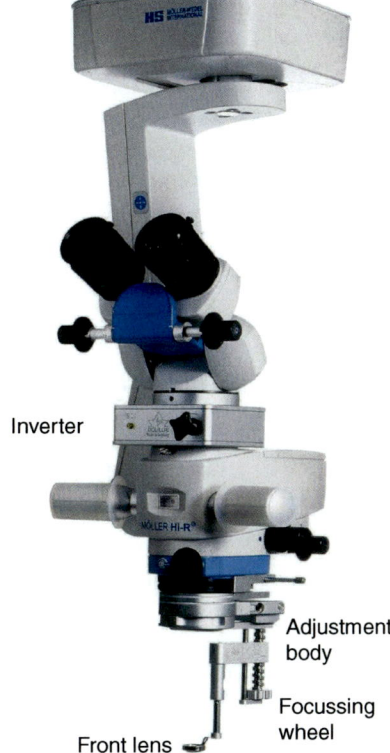

Inverter

Adjustment body

Focussing wheel

Front lens

Remember following steps:

1. Minimal zoom.
2. Turn the BIOM-adjustment body with the focus wheel to the top position.
3. Move the microscope with the focus foot pedal so far down towards the cornea, until you get a fairly big image (red pupil).
4. Turn the focus wheel (BIOM) until you get a sharp retinal image.

If the image is sharp, move the microscope further down towards the cornea with the focus of the foot pedal (Careful of corneal touch!). Lastly, you can increase the zoom with the zoom pedal but be aware that the resolution decreases the more zoom you have. If the image is totally blurred and you eventually cannot continue, or you changed the front lens, always return to the initial parameters (lowest zoom, BIOM adjustment body to the top). Remark: Bringing the microscope focus down gives you a wider field increasing the zoom gives you a magnified view.

If you are using the *Resight* system, there is only one adjustable wheel at the viewing system. Minimize the zoom of the microscope with the foot pedal, flick in the Resight viewing system, activate the inverter and then turn the wheel at the viewing system until the image is sharp.

If you are using the *RUV800 or Eibos* system, try to reach the manual focus with your right index or middle finger. Once you have mastered this, it makes focusing a lot easier than advising the scrub nurse in focusing up or down. The RUV800 or Eibos system is the easiest-to-use of all viewing systems.

Important It may happen that the view to fundus is poor. The reason is media opacities. Hold the vitreous cutter behind the lens capsule. Is the vitreous cutter sharp and focused? If yes, then an opacity of the vitreous is present. If no, then a media opacity of the cornea, anterior chamber or lens must be present. In latter case, you can perform a corneal abrasion, remove blood or fibrin from the anterior chamber and perform a phacoemulsification in case of a mature cataract.

Tips and Tricks
Corneal lubrication: A major problem during vitrectomy, especially in combined surgeries with a duration of over 1 hour, is corneal epithelial edema. With the application of methylcellulose (Celoftal®, Alcon or Ocucoat®, Bausch&Lomb) on the cornea the cornea can remain clear for many hours. A debridement of the epithelium is rarely necessary, but if needed use a broad blade (crescent knife).

Tips and Tricks
Small pupil: If the pupil contracts during surgery, inject 0.01% adrenaline into the anterior chamber. The pupil should enlarge within seconds. If the small pupil is caused by posterior synechiae use stretching instruments such as a Sinskey hook or insert iris hooks to enlarge the pupil.

Tips and Tricks
BIOM and air: If you perform a water against air exchange the image will become blurred. You can focus the image by turning the focus wheel of the BIOM so that the front lens moves up. The image will become focused again.

5. Core vitrectomy

Now we start at last with the vitrectomy. You start with the core vitrectomy. In contrast to cataract surgery, you will be surprised by how much space you have in the vitreous cavity. The core vitreous is removed in two steps. First the temporal (or nasal) half is removed, then the instruments are switched, and the other half is removed.

In contrast to phacoemulsification where you hold the instruments almost horizontal, you hold the instruments during vitrectomy almost perpendicular (towards the optic nerve) (Fig. 24.6).

Make calm and slow movements with the vitreous cutter; this is in contrast to irrigation/aspiration during phaco. Another important difference is that you hardly move the irrigation handpiece during phaco, but the light pipe in vitrectomy is in constant motion. Light pipe and vitreous cutter move simultaneously, the light pipe illuminating the path of the vitreous cutter. You point the beam of the light pipe to the tip of the vitreous cutter.

The main problem of vitrectomy is the poor visibility of the transparent vitreous. You recognize the vitreous best in the light cone. For visualization of the vitreous hold the light pipe close to the vitreous cutter. You see the vitreous like holding a torch light into a smoke stack.

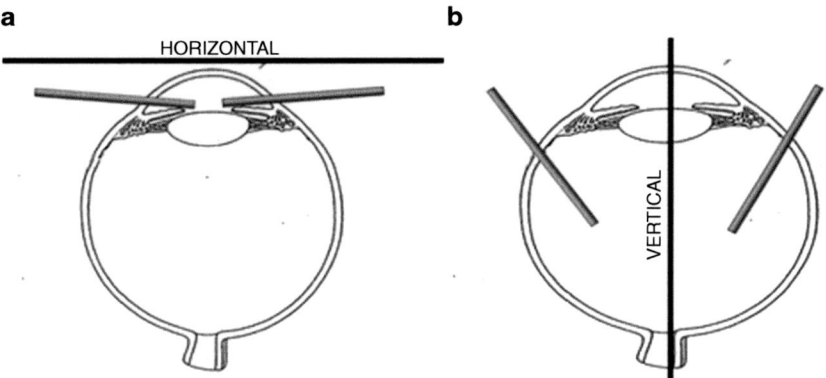

Fig. 24.6 (**a**) In cataract surgery the instruments are held almost *horizontal*. (**b**) In vitreoretinal surgery the Instruments are held almost *vertical*

Table 24.2 Approximate settings for small gauge with different vitrectomy machines

	Old generation vitrectomy machines with 2500 cpm		Infinity phacoemulsification machine with 2500 cpm	
	Cutting speed cpm	Vacuum mm Hg	Cutting speed cpm	Vacuum mm Hg
Core vitrectomy	1500	400	2500	500–600
PVD	0	400–600	0	Maximal vacuum (650 mmHg)
Peripheral vitrectomy	2500	0–200	2500	200–300
Opening of posterior capsule	400	400	500	300

PVD posterior vitreous detachment, *cpm* cuts per minute

In eyes with synchisis scintillans or asteroid hyalosis the vitreous can be seen very clearly. As a beginner stain the vitreous body during your first surgeries with triamcinolone.

Move both instruments in a half circle in the vitreous cavity as if peeling an onion from inside to outside. The nasal vitreous is cut with the vitrector from the temporal trocar cannula and the temporal vitreous is removed from the nasal trocar cannula.

Be cautious, if you come close to the retina with the vitreous cutter. You can estimate the vicinity to the retina by looking at the shadow of the vitreous cutter. Be aware: The retina forgives no mistakes, and retinal breaks are made quickly.

The settings for the vitrectomy machine can be adjusted according to the individual preferences and the vitrectomy machine. For details see Table 24.2.

The settings for an phacoemulsification machine are depicted in Fig. 24.7.

It is also important to clear the vitreous immediately in front of your ports. Otherwise, there is the danger of pushing the vitreous base forward when introduc-

Fig. 24.7 Settings for vitrectomy with an Infinity phacoemulsification machine. Note continuous irrigation, I/A-cut and cutting speed of 2500 cuts/min. The infusion pressure is reduced to 45 cmH$_2$O (= 33 mmHg)

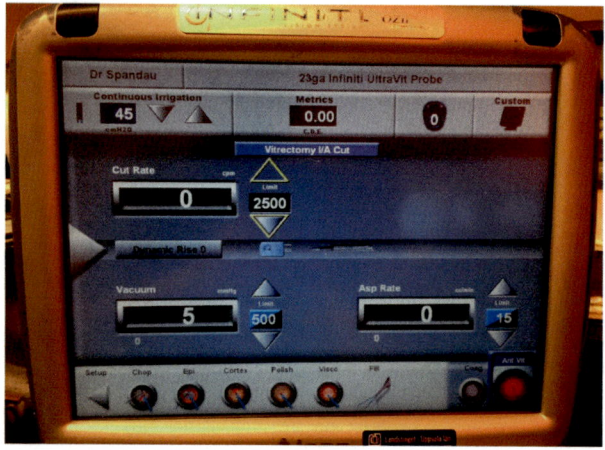

ing your instruments, thereby causing retinal breaks in the vitreous base. This is of particular importance when introducing blunt instruments, for example, a flute needle or an injection cannula.

Tips and Tricks

Subepithelial location of infusion cannula: Even an initially correctly placed trocar cannula may move subepithelial during a later stage of the operation. If you experience a retinal or choroidal detachment, stop the infusion, remove the infusion line and insert it in an area without choroidal detachment. Re-open the infusion and the retina or choroid will reattach. Now check the location of the infusion cannula. Is it 3.5 mm posterior the limbus? If not, replace the trocar cannula correctly. Is the trocar located subepithelial? If so, then free the trocar from the tissue with a membrane pic inserted in the opposite cannula.

6. Induction of posterior vitreous detachment (Fig. 24.8)

For this step, we routinely use a 90D front lens. To induce a posterior vitreous detachment is a difficult procedure in the learning phase. We recommend beginners to stain the posterior pole at the beginning of vitrectomy with trypan blue. The vitreous is much easier to recognize and especially the induction of a posterior vitreous detachment become considerably easier. Inject a small amount of trypan blue that will drop down onto the posterior pole. Do not inject too much trypan blue. The dye will very nicely stain the bursa praemacularis of the vitreous. The bursa praemacularis is a cavity anterior to the macula.

For induction of PVD, position the vitreous cutter at the nasal rim of the optic disc with the aspiration port pointing to the ora serrata. Then increase suction (foot pedal to bottom position) to a maximum. In the suction phase the vitreous cortex and especially the posterior hyaloid will be engaged in the aspiration port. Then draw the vitreous cutter slowly with maximal suction towards the lens. If the maneuver is successful, you will see a kind of fine silk screen that moves forward together with the vitreous cutter. Try to keep an eye on the advancing posterior vitreous face

Fig. 24.8 Induction of
PVD. Place the tip of the
cutter at the nasal edge of
the optic disc. Aspirate
maximal, the vitreous
cortex engages in the cutter
opening and then pull the
cutter slowly forward

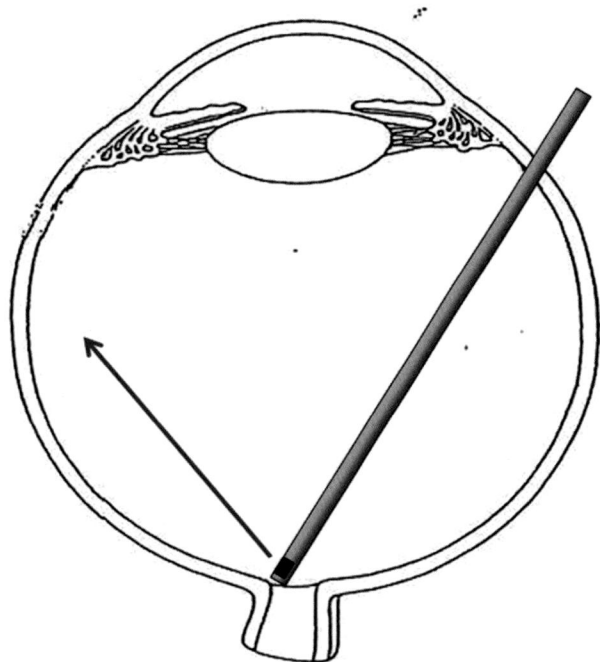

in the mid-periphery. This looks like a tidal wave. It is where breaks will develop
during induction of a PVD. Sometimes, this whole maneuver must be repeated several times until it succeeds. Before you repeat the maneuver cut the aspirated vitreous in the vitreous cutter to prevent traction and tractional tears and then place the
vitreous cutter in front of the optic disc again.

Remark: If you are using a *phacoemulsification* machine then perform a PVD in the
I/A setting and maximal vaccum. Press the foot pedal so that you are in the I/A step.

7. Removal of peripheral vitreous

After successful PVD, continue with removal of peripheral vitreous. We usually
use a 120D or comparable wide-angle lens. Regarding the settings of the vitrectomy
machine, decrease the vacuum and increase the cutting frequency the closer to retina you work with the vitrector (Table 24.2).

In phakic eyes, you can cross the midline only when working at the posterior
pole to mid-periphery. To reach the vitreous base, you are not allowed to cross the
midline. The vitreous base can be removed from the opposite site by indenting the
vitreous base.

Tips and Tricks
Working in the area of the vitreous base and *trimming the vitreous base* is another
key step to learn if you want to master vitrectomy. Numerous techniques can be
used. Our favourite technique is using a chandelier light and indentation with a
scleral depressor.

Tips and Tricks

Scleral folds or soft globe during vitrectomy: If you view scleral folds during vitrectomy or if the globe is soft, then stop PPV at once. The most likely cause is a dislocated infusion line. Reinsert the infusion line and check if the globe is normotensive and if the scleral folds have vanished.

8. Internal search for retinal breaks

At the end of vitrectomy breaks must be identified and treated accordingly. Inspect the entire peripheral retina with the aid of a scleral depressor. If a break is present, you must remove any residual vitreous adhesions, treat the break with laser- or cryoretinopexy and a gas tamponade needs to be accomplished. Alternatively to a gas injection you can inject 0,5 ml air into the vitreous cavity after removal of all trocars. Otherwise a postoperative retinal detachment occurs.

Tips and Tricks

Internal search for retinal breaks: Perform an internal search in each and every case of vitrectomy, even in low-risk cases. Perform the search at the very end of your procedure, as even minor intraocular manipulations may create breaks in the area of the vitreous base that may not be noticed if you have performed your inspection of the vitreous base beforehand.

Tips and Tricks

Iatrogenic break: When a small break is located within the vascular arcades, a laser treatment is not necessary as the pigment epithelium in the central area has sufficient pumping function so that no detachment occurs. If the break is large, however, we recommend lasering the break with one row of laser burns. Even if you create a peripheral break this is not a problem as long as you also recognize the break. Surround the tear with three rows of laser burns and perform a gas or air tamponade.

9. Laser therapy

A laser treatment can be carried out in a water- (BSS)-filled, silicone oil filled and PFCL-filled eye. In an air-filled eye, it is difficult to laser due to a poor visibility.

It is easiest to laser breaks under heavy liquid (PFCL), as you have a good apposition of retina and retinal pigment epithelium. One of the disadvantages of this technique is that the margins of the break are more difficult to see. Mark, therefore, the location of breaks with endodiathermy or laser spots before covering it with heavy liquid. This way it is easy to identify them under heavy liquid.

The further you move the laser probe away from the retina, the larger the resulting spot size on the retina (and the more energy you need to create a burn). This can be quite useful if you want to treat larger areas as the resulting burns have softer edges and do not cut the retina like a knife.

Use 360° prophylactic laser with caution. It may not be necessary, may result in anterior segment ischemia and will make it very difficult to identify small breaks in cases of postoperative retinal detachments.

10. Cryotherapy of peripheral break

The cryotherapy of a peripheral break is a good alternative to laser photocoagulation, in particular in phakic eye where endolaser of breaks in the retinal periphery without touching the lens is challenging. You indent the retina with the cryo probe and hold the light pipe in the other hand. Cryotherapy should be applied sparingly, preferably with one cryo effect in the middle of the break in order to reduce the risk for PVR. Cryotherapy induces more PVR than laser photocoagulation due to greater breakdown of the blood retinal barrier.

11. Intraoperative Tamponade (short term tamponade)

During vitrectomy, an intraoperative tamponade with perfluorocarbon (PFCL) or air is performed. There are several indications. A fluid against air exchange is an important step in detachment surgery. A PFCL (heavy liquid) tamponade is important to attach a detached retina or elevate a dropped nucleus. PFCL must always be completely removed because it damages the retina. It is very important to know the physiologic properties of PFCL and air (Fig. 24.9).

The following instruments and cannulas are required for injection of PFCL and air: (1) Charles flute handpiece and canula (backflush instrument) (Figs. 24.10, 24.11, 24.12) and a (2) dual bore cannula (Fig. 24.13).

Fig. 24.9 Opposite effects of air and PFCL in the vitreous cavity. Air exerts pressure onto the retina from anterior to posterior whereas PFCL exerts pressure from posterior to anterior

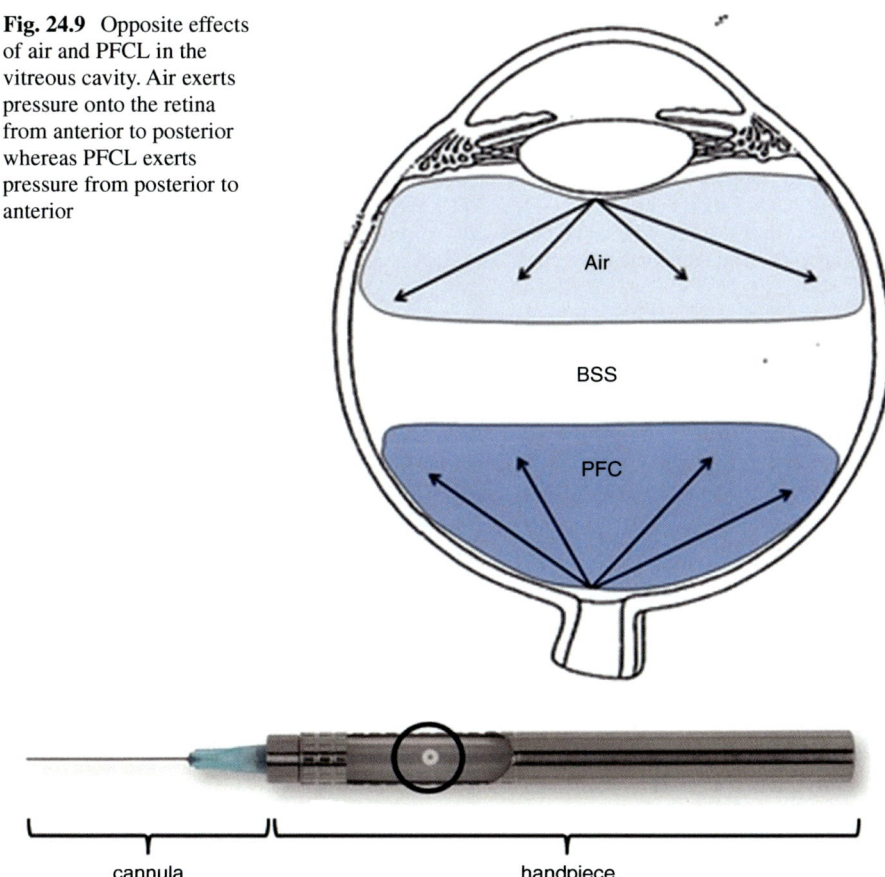

Fig. 24.10 The Charles flute needle aspirates fluid through the needle on the left side and the water flows out through the hole in the middle (circle). This is called *passive aspiration*

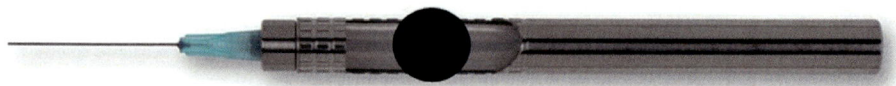

Fig. 24.11 If you close the hole at the side with your index finger then the Charles flute needle does not aspirate. You do not need to press the tubing but only close the hole

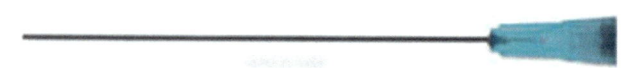

Fig 24.12 23-Gauge backflush (Charles) needle. This cannula is used for the flute *instrument and for injection of fluids. If you inject a fluid into the eye, you need to release* fluid at the same time from the eye. This is done bimanual with a Charles flute handpiece (backflush needle). A chandelier light is required. DORC 1281.A5D06

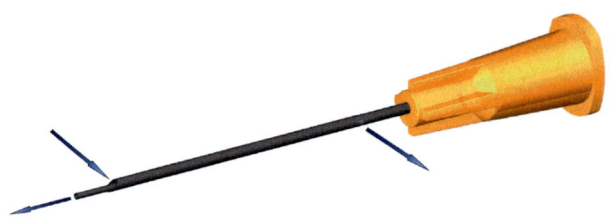

Fig 24.13 Double-barreled (dual bore) cannula. This cannula is used for the injection of heavy fluid (PFCL). This special cannula injects PFCL into the eye and at the same time fluid passively egresses from the eye. The cannula prevents an intraocular hypertension during injection. The injection is done monomanual, a chandelier light is not required. DORC: Double bore cannula. EFD.06

Function of Charles flute handpiece (backflush instrument) (Figs. 24.10 and 24.11).

PFCL Injection (Fig. 24.14)
Inject PFCL always in a fluid filled eye and not in an air-filled eye. The PFCL must be injected slowly. PFCL injected too quickly can induce retinal damage. PFCL should <u>never</u> be injected in direction of the macula. You start with the injection nasal to the optic disc and then move the cannula slowly towards the lens leaving the tip of the cannula in the PFCL bubble. Leaving the tip of the cannula in the big bubble prevents the formation of small PFCL bubbles (fish eggs). PFCL can be injected (1) bimanual with a Charles flute cannula. At the same time, BSS is released with a backflush instrument. A chandelier light is therefore needed (Fig. 24.14a). (2) monomanual with a dual bore cannula which allows simultaneous injection and decompression (Fig. 24.14b).

Tips and Tricks
Observe the venous pulsation of the disc vessels while injecting PFCL.

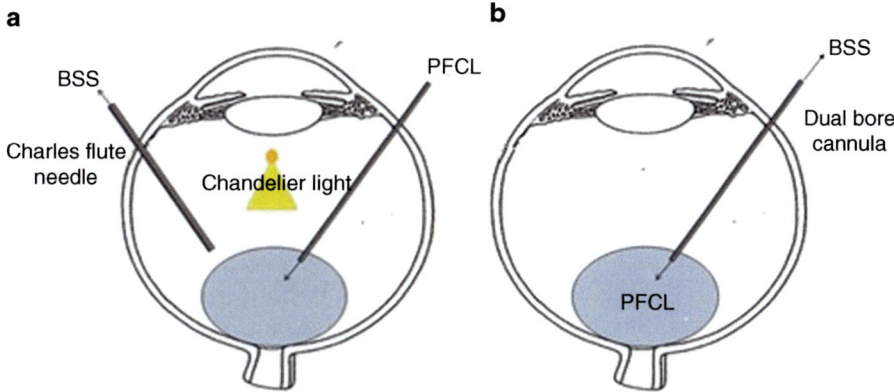

Fig. 24.14 (**a**) Bimanual injection of PFCL with Charles flute cannula. At the same time BSS is removed with a second extrusion cannula. A chandelier light is required. (**b**) Monomanual injection of PFCL with a dual bore cannula. The cannula injects PFCL as well as removes BSS at the same time. A chandelier light is *not* required

Removal of PFCL
Hold the flute needle in front of the optic disc and aspirate the complete PFCL bubble. If a small bubble remain and you do not succeed with the flute needle, then do not insist but aspirate the residual bubble with a silicone tip flute needle in order not to damage the retina or the optic disc.

12. Postoperative Tamponade (long term tamponade)

A long-term tamponade is gas (air, Sf_6, C_2F_6 and C_3F_8) or a silicone oil. In easy cases an air tamponade is sufficient. Before injecting the long term tamponade, a fluid against air exchange (FAX) is performed.

Fluid Against Air Exchange (FAX)
Fluid x air exchange means fluid against air exchange. During this maneuver the BSS inside the vitreous cavity is exchanged against air. This is a very common surgical maneuver during vitreoretinal surgery and at the end of vitreoretinal surgery. At the end of vitreoretinal surgery, the air may be used as tamponade or be exchanged against a longer lasting gas such as Sf_6, C_2F_6 and C_3F_8. A fluid against air exchange is performed with a Charles flute needle (= backflush instrument) (Fig. 24.10). Place the tip of the flute needle close to the posterior pole and switch from fluid to air. Then wait until the air reaches the posterior pole.

An air tamponade has several indications: (1) Air in the vitreous cavity presses against the wedges of the sclerotomy incision and thereby stabilizes the sclerotomies, which results in a reduced postoperative hypotony.(2) Reduces postoperative bleeding (favourable for diabetic eyes). (3) Can act as weak and short-term tamponade.

Remark: For a fluid x air exchange a fluid/air pump is required. This pump is not integrated in a phacoemulsification machine.

13. Removal of the trocar cannulas

It is useful to remove the trocars in the following order: first the instrument trocars, then the chandelier light, and finally the infusion cannula. The infusion cannula remains in place until the end to avoid hypotension when removing the trocars. The infusion should therefore remain open until removal of the infusion cannula. To remove the trocars, pull out the trocar with the trocar forceps, then press the edges of the sclerotomy together with the forceps. Lastly the infusion cannula is removed. Before you do this, check the intraocular pressure manually. If you observe uveal tissue or even a vitreous prolapse out of the sclerotomy you should remove it with the vitreous cutter because otherwise there is a possible wicking and endophthalmitis risk. If the sclerotomy is still leaking, it should be closed with a suture. The sclerotomy should be covered by conjunctiva; otherwise it is recommended that the sclerotomy be sutured.A major advantage of not suturing a gas filled eye is the prevention of IOP spikes in the postoperative course, as the expanding gas can escape postoperatively through the non-sutured sclerotomies.

Tips and Tricks

Sclerotomy
(1) For beginners, we recommend opening the conjunctiva in the area of the sclerotomies in order to recognize the sclerotomies clearly. This is particularly important if you want to suture the sclerotomy at the end of the procedure.
(2) In the case of doubt, suture the sclerotomy. The potential disadvantages of a leaking sclerotomy outweigh the discomfort of a single suture.

14. Sclerotomy sutures

A 23-Gauge sclerotomy can be sutured with an 8–0 Vicryl simple interrupted stitch and a 20-Gauge-sclerotomy with a Vicryl 8–0 cross stitch. To suture a sclerotomy is harder than you assume. Grasp one edge of the sclerotomy with surgical forceps, move the needle through the sclerotomy edge, then grasp the opposite edge of the sclerotomy with the forceps and pull the needle through the second edge. In case of a 20G sclerotomy a X-suture (Vicryl 8–0) is required; for a 23G sclerotomy a single interrupted stitch is sufficient. Test with the swab whether the sclerotomy is closed. If it still leaks, remove the suture and place a new suture.

Tips and Tricks

Leaking Sclerotomies
(1) A leak can be identified by a chemotic conjunctiva above the sclerotomy in a fluid filled eye or by air bubbles in an air-filled eye. If the sclerotomies leak, then place a Vicryl 8–0 simple interrupted stitch on the sclerotomy (Fig. 24.15).
(2) These can occur after multiple vitrectomies and a large opening, for example, for silicone oil removal or if multiple sclerotomies have been placed in the same location. It is not uncommon in high myopes with a thin sclera. To close these

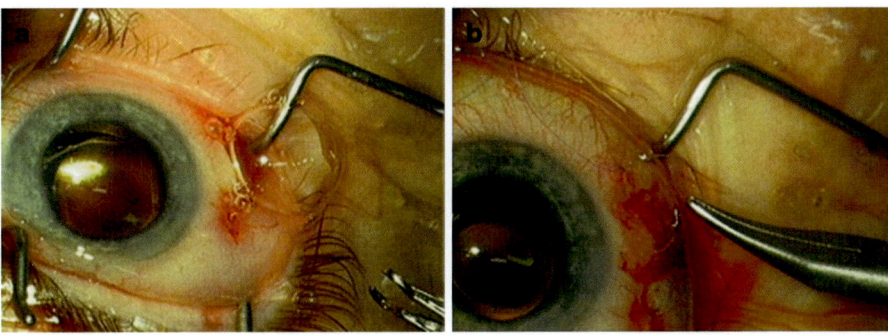

Fig 24.15 (**a**) Leakage of air from a sclerotomy in an eye with air tamponade. In this case the sclerotomy should be sutured. (**b**) After suturing the sclerotomy with a Vicryl 8-0 simple interrupted stitch the sclerotomy is closed airtight

large sclerotomies, do not use multiple single sutures (they make it worse) or large sutures (the larger needles may cause additional holes in the sclera). Place a 7-0 or 8-0 Vicryl cross stitch on the sclerotomy. Stay very superficially within the sclera and do not go "deep". Use a long intrascleral path. Finally, use 4 instead of 3 throws for your first knot and ask the scrub nurse to close the infusion temporarily while you tighten the knot.

Postoperative Treatment for Conventional Vitrectomy Combined Dexamethasone-Gentamicin drops 5x daily for 2 weeks and 3x daily for third week. Then stop. Atropine drops 1x daily for 2 weeks.

The Videos 24.1, 24.2, 24.3, 24.4, 24.5, and 24.6 demonstrate the surgical management of interesting anterior segment pathologies.

A Materials and Companies

A. 1 Materials (in Alphabetical order)

AUROLAB
- No: 1, Sivagangai Main Road
- Veerapanjan, Madurai, 625 020, Tamil Nadu, India.
- Phone : + 91 – 452 – 2446100
- Fax : + 91 – 452 – 2446200c
- Website: http://aurolab.com

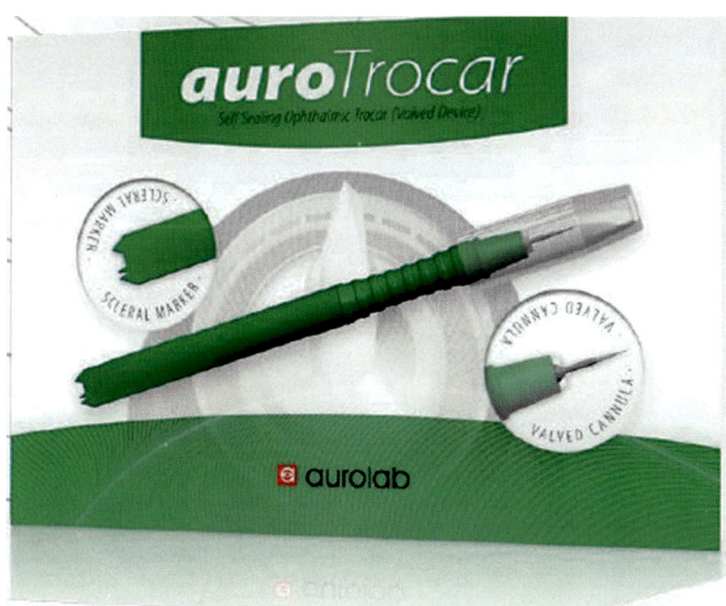

A one-step trocar (23G) set with infusion line. Aurolab, India

© Springer Nature Switzerland AG 2020
U. Spandau, *Trocar Surgery for Cataract Surgeons*,
https://doi.org/10.1007/978-3-030-36093-1

DORC
- D.O.R.C. Germany GmbH
- Charlottenstr. 80
- 10117 Berlin
- Phone: 030/20188364
- Fax: 030/20188365
- Website: https://DORC.nl

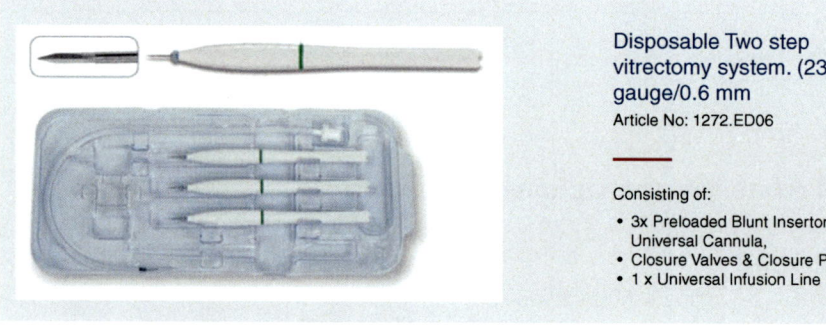

Disposable Two step vitrectomy system. (23 gauge/0.6 mm
Article No: 1272.ED06

Consisting of:
- 3x Preloaded Blunt Insertor with Universal Cannula,
- Closure Valves & Closure Plugs
- 1 x Universal Infusion Line

A one step trocar (23G) set with infusion line. DORC, Netherlands

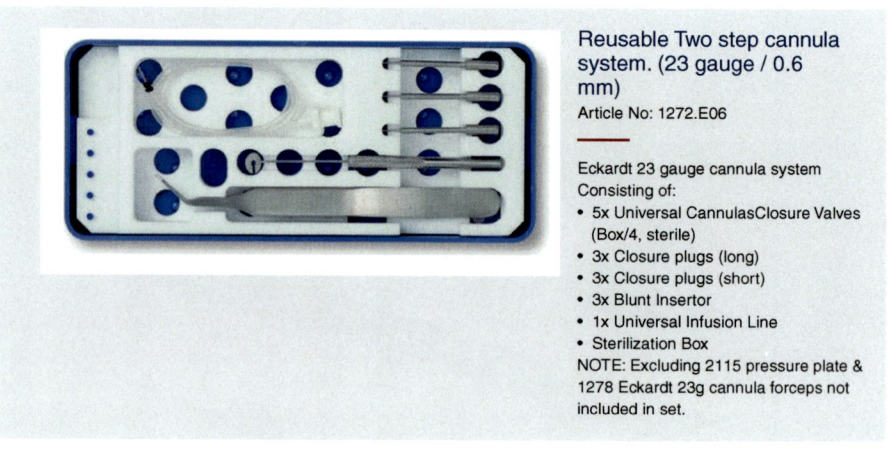

Reusable Two step cannula system. (23 gauge / 0.6 mm)
Article No: 1272.E06

Eckardt 23 gauge cannula system
Consisting of:
- 5x Universal CannulasClosure Valves (Box/4, sterile)
- 3x Closure plugs (long)
- 3x Closure plugs (short)
- 3x Blunt Insertor
- 1x Universal Infusion Line
- Sterilization Box
NOTE: Excluding 2115 pressure plate & 1278 Eckardt 23g cannula forceps not included in set.

A reusable trocar (23G) set with infusion line. DORC, Netherlands

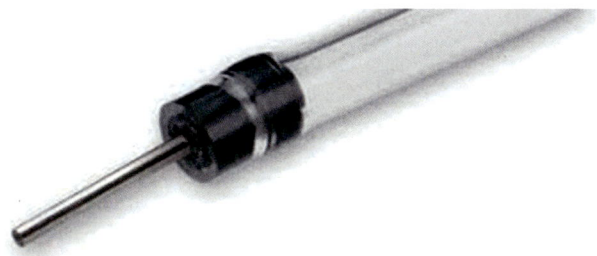

Infusion line (23G, DORC, No: 1279.VFI.)

FCI

- **FCI** sells vitreoretinal equipment. Trocars, light fibers, instruments
- FCI S.A.S. – France Chirurgie Instrumentation
- 20-22 rue Louis Armand
- 75015 PARIS – France
- Phone: +33 1 53 98 98 97
- Fax: +33 1 53 98 98 99
- Website: https://fciworldwide.com

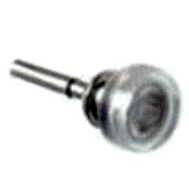
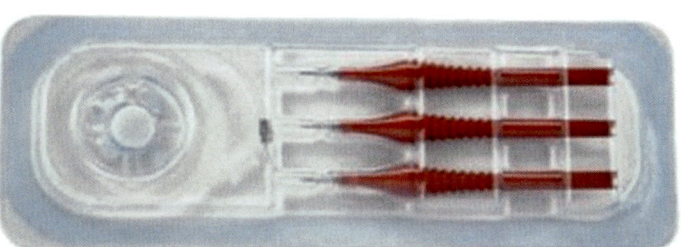
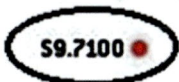

A one step trocar (23G) set with infusion line. FCI, France

MANI

Manufacturer :

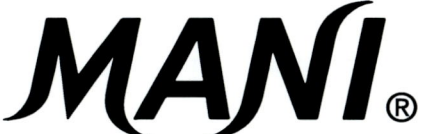

8-3 Kiyohara Industrial Park,
Utsunomiya, Tochigi, 321-3231 JAPAN
TEL: +81.28.667.7565 / FAX: +81.28.667.8305
URL: http://www.mani.co.jp/en/
E-mail: seg-ovs@ms.mani.co.jp

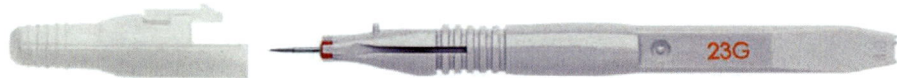

A single trocar (23G) from Mani, Japan

- Trocar blade in the shape of MVR knife.
- Ultimate sharpness adopting proven technologies of MANI® Ophthalmic Knife.
- Valved cannula for the simpler operation.
- Sterile individual pack (1 pc.) for additional requirement or backup.

Product Name	Packaging	Color Coding	Order #
Trocar 25G S	6 Pcs. / Box		MTR25S
Trocar 23G S	6 Pcs. / Box		MTR23S

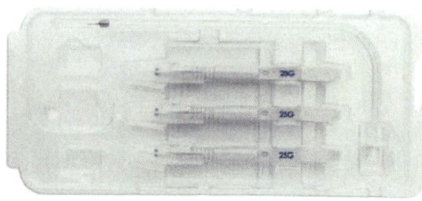

Product Name	Packaging	Order #
Trocar Kit 25G S	3 Kits / Box	MTK25S
Trocar Kit 23G S	3 Kits / Box	MTK23S

- Sterile 1 Kit consists of 3 pcs. trocar with the valved cannula and 1 pc. infusion cannula.

A one step trocar (23G) set with infusion line. Mani, Japan

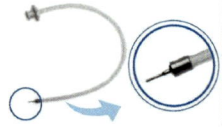 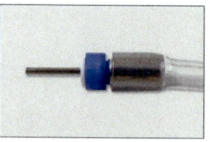

Connection with the valved cannula

Product Name	Packaging	Order #
Infusion Cannula 25G S	6 Pcs. / Box	MIC25S
Infusion Cannula 23G S	6 Pcs. / Box	MIC23S

- Attaching directly to the valved cannula.
- Sterile individual pack (1 pc.) for additional requirement or backup.

23G infusion line from Mani, Inc (Japan)
Website: http://www.mani.co.jp/en/product/ophthalmic.html#

A. 2 Other Companies Selling Vitreoretinal Products (in Alphabetical Order)

Advanced Visual Instruments, Inc.(sells contact lenses for vitrectomy)
- 411, 5th Avenue 4th Floor
- New York, NY 10016
- Phone: (212) 262 – 7878
- Fax: 1-973-625-8237
- e-mail: https://avig@avi-panoramic.com

Beaver-Visitec International, Ltd (sells anterior segment equipment)
- Centurion Court
- 85c Milton Park
- Abingdon, Oxfordshire
- OX14 4RY

- UK
- Website: www.Beaver-Visitec.com

CROMA GmbH (sells viscoelastics and products for anterior and posterior segment)
- Industrial Line 6
- 2100 Leobendorf
- Austria
- Phone: +43/2262/684680

Eye Technology Ltd. (Sells vitreoretinal instruments)
- 19 Totman Crescent
- Brook Road Industrial Estate
- Rayleigh
- Essex SS6 7UY
- United Kingdom
- e-mail: https://sales@eye-tech.co.uk

Fluoron GmbH (sells intraocular fluids such as Densiron 68)
- Magirus-Deutz-Straße 10
- 89077 Ulm
- Phone: 0731/20559970
- Fax: 0731/205 599 728
- e-mail: https://info@fluoron.de
- Website: www.fluoron.de

Geuder (sells anterior segment and vitreoretinal instruments)
- Hertzstr. 4
- 69126 Heidelberg
- Phone: 06221/3066
- Fax: 06221/303122
- e-mail: https://info@geuder.de
- Website: www.geuder.de

Madhu industries
- A-260, Okhla Industrial Area Phase - 1,
- New Delhi – 110020, India
- Website: https://www.madhuinstruments.com

Medone Surgical Inc. (sells vitreoretinal equipment)
- Sarasota, FL 34243
- USA
- Website: www.MedOne.com

Ocular Instruments (sell contact lenses for vitrectomy)
- 2255 116th Ave NE, Bellevue,
- Washington 98004-3039
- USA

- Phone: 425-455-5200 or 800-888-6616
- Fax: 425-462-6669
- e-mail: https://ocular@ocularinc.com
- Website: www.ocularinc.com

Oculus Optic device GmbH (sells BIOM and lenses)
- Münchholzhäuser Strasse 29
- D-35582 Wetzlar
- Germany
- Phone: 0641/20050
- Fax: 0641/2005255
- e-mail: https://sales@oculus.de
- Website: www.oculus.de

Opthec BV (sells Artisan and pigmented IOL)
- Schweitzerlaan 15
- 9728 NR Groningen
- Netherlands
- Phone: +31 050 5251944
- Website: www.opthec.com

Synergetics (sells trocars, light fibers, instruments)
- Synergetics Germany GmbH Körnerstraße 59
- 58095 Hagen
- Phone: 0641/20050
- Fax: 0641/2005255
- e-mail: https://blangohr@synergeticsusa.com
- Website: www.synergeticsusa.com

Index

© Springer Nature Switzerland AG 2020
U. Spandau, *Trocar Surgery for Cataract Surgeons*,
https://doi.org/10.1007/978-3-030-36093-1

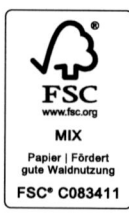

Zeitfracht Medien GmbH
Ferdinand-Jühlke-Straße 7
99095 Erfurt, Deutschland
produktsicherheit@kolibri360.de